D0497271

COMMANDO
WORKOUT

COMMANDO
WORKOUT

4 weeks to total fitness

**Simon
Waterson**

with
Sally Brown

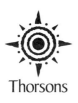

Thorsons

Thorsons
An Imprint of HarperCollins*Publishers*
77–85 Fulham Palace Road
Hammersmith, London W6 8JB

The Thorsons website address is:
www.thorsons.com

and *Thorsons* are trademarks of
HarperCollins*Publishers* Limited

First published by Thorsons 2002

1 3 5 7 9 10 8 6 4 2

© Simon Waterson, 2002

Simon Waterson asserts the moral right to
be identified as the author of this work

A catalogue record of this book
is available from the British Library

ISBN 0 00 714297 8

Photography by Robin Matthews

Printed and bound in Great Britain by
Scotprint, Haddington, East Lothian

All rights reserved. No part of this publication may be
reproduced, stored in a retrieval system, or transmitted,
in any form or by any means, electronic, mechanical,
photocopying, recording or otherwise, without the prior
written permission of the publishers.

CONTENTS

GOING COMMANDO

Commandos are the fitness elite of the military. They are in peak physical condition at all times, ready to go into action at short notice and to deal with crisis situations in some of the most world's most extreme physical and climatic terrain. Men from the ground, sea and air forces can put themselves forward for commando training, but to be accepted you must pass one of the most gruelling tests of fitness and mental strength known to the Western world. If you succeed, you've earned the right to wear the coveted Green Beret insignia that brings with it the respect of fighting forces around the world.

I went through basic military training at age 16. Then, after passing the first 2 stages of the British Royal Navy training, I elected to join a Naval Air Commando squadron. Having spent time training with the Royal Navy, I thought that I'd seen it all – but the commando course was a whole new level of endurance training. The pass rate for commando training is low, with just 16–20% of hopefuls making the grade.

On an average day, you might do a 7-mile 'yomp' (a mix of fast walking and running) across rough terrain with a full pack on your back, followed by a timed assault course and then target shooting. To top it all, you may have to hold your weapon in one hand straight out from your body for 3 minutes. Any tests you fail are punished with press-ups, sit-ups or a 100m sprint with your mate over your shoulder. And it all has to be completed with immaculate kit and personal appearance at all times.

At 16, I was 10 stone and considered myself fit. By the time I had completed my commando training, I was 14 stone of pure muscle and could run 7-minute miles and do 100 metres in 11 seconds. I thought nothing of signing up for events like the Royal Tournament Field Gun Competition, which involves running with a 1-ton gun as part of an 18-man team, or running a half marathon for fun at the weekend.

SECRETS OF THE COMMANDO TRAINING TECHNIQUE

As a commando, once you have passed the initial training course, keeping yourself in peak condition becomes your own responsibility – there is no training team to shout you out of bed at 5am when you need to go do a 6-mile run with a heavy rucksack on your back. It is expected that you are committed and will fit your training into the working day, whatever your circumstances. But what commandos have to help them, thanks to specific training methods, are the skills and attitude to motivate themselves to maintain their physical fitness – wherever they are in the world and however little time they have spare. Everyone has the ability to learn and develop these motivational and training skills.

A commando is taught a training technique that is so effective that it is possible to maintain a high level of fitness in just 30 minutes a day – without needing a gym or any specialist equipment. The commando's workout must be simple, flexible and effective – and challenging!

★ **Simple.** Experience in the field shows that keeping it simple gets the best results when the going gets tough. Keeping it simple also means that it is easier to focus on your goals and do the right thing without confusing your mind or body.

★ **Flexible.** Commandos learn how to adapt and improvise – to make the best of any situation. This makes for a flexible attitude to training so there is less chance of anything getting in the way of fitness. A flexible attitude means you'll find fewer excuses for sticking to your workout plans.

★ **Effective.** Commando techniques for developing strength and stamina have been fine-tuned over the years to produce a system that's unbeatable for effectiveness and reliability.

The training sessions are designed to challenge the body and mind, and consist of both cardiovascular and strength-training activities – both based on the principle of interval training. Exercise gets results when it places stress on the body – or 'overload' as it's known technically – forcing it to make adaptations to make itself stronger. By overloading the body on a regular basis, the heart and lungs become more efficient at delivering oxygen and eliminating waste products and the muscle cells become more efficient at burning fuel. But the human body cannot tolerate working at the extreme edge of its capabilities for any sustained period, so this is where interval training comes in – combining bouts of high intensity with periods of recovery within the same session. This allows you to push yourself hard enough to challenge your body without the risk of injury.

This 'on-off' system of working out is no cop-out or cheat's option. In fact, it's the intelligent approach to reaching better levels of fitness and is the system guaranteed to get the best results.

In addition, the routine not only improves muscular strength but also endurance and stamina. Being able to lift a very heavy weight just once might be impressive in the gym but it is not practical in the field or in everyday life where you need to be able to perform strenuous activities over and over again. The commando emphasis on a combination of strength training and endurance work is one of the keys to the outstanding abilities of our soldiers in the field. It can mean the difference between life and death – if a colleague is injured, you have to be capable of carrying him for miles to get help. You are only as fast and effective as your slowest man – that is why it is important to stay fit as you are all reliant on each other.

But you don't need to join the armed forces to benefit from well-balanced fitness and an effective workout routine. If you are interested in feeling fitter, stronger, more alert and alive, and in improving your self-discipline and mental attitude, then the commando workout system will meet your needs and help you reach your personal goals – whatever they may be.

This style of training also develops 'functional fitness'. If your only form of exercise is working out on gym equipment such as treadmills and weight training machines, no matter how dedicated you are, your body will only ever be efficient at working out on those machines; your muscles will adapt to a very specific and limited type of work. But if your exercise routine involves working with your own bodyweight as resistance, you are recruiting and forcing every muscle into action and improving core strength and balance into the bargain. For instance, use a triceps pushdown machine in the gym and your tricep muscle is isolated and targeted. Exercise your triceps muscles by doing close-arm press-ups and you are also targeting the pectorals, deltoids and triceps (chest, shoulder and back of arm muscles), as well as improving your core strength by using hundreds of vital secondary muscles to stabilise your body during the movement. You are teaching your muscles to work together and the end result is a more balanced body – in terms of appearance and function – and a more efficient one.

HOW THE COMMANDO WORKOUT WILL WORK FOR YOU

The core principles of the Commando Workout will benefit anyone who genuinely desires to improve their physical and mental condition. Modelled on the approach used to take soldiers to new levels of strength and fitness, this program is specifically designed for use by ordinary civilians from all walks of life. Each of us has the potential to find new strength, confidence and motivation and it's my plan to take you there!

The Commando Workout is an effort-based program, which means it is designed to suit anyone of any fitness level. If you are already a regular exerciser, don't assume that a program that can be done by beginners won't be 'hard' enough for you. If you work out several times a week and feel you've reached an exercise plateau, this is *definitely* the program for you.

Since the program is effort-based, the ground rule is that at all times you do *your* best. When the program calls for light effort, you cruise, but when it calls for flat-out hard work, you go for it – as hard as you can. By using interval training in this way, you are guaranteed to see a change no matter what your starting point.

Your results will be as large or small as you want them to be, and they will be different for every person. But what you will all see is a drop in body fat and an increase in lean muscle tissue. Your heart will pump more blood around your body, your lungs will extract oxygen from the bloodstream more effectively and you'll have increased muscular strength and endurance. But the changes aren't just physical; a commando also needs to be quick thinking, alert and happy. The 4-week program will test you as a person. It is hard work, but the largest gain is self-discipline. Exercise will become a breeze because of the mental strength you will have gained. Be prepared for the biggest change of your life.

Over the 4 weeks, you will lose weight. But this program is about achieving much more than that so don't make this your only goal or focus. Equally important is that you will experience:

★ Increased cardiovascular (heart and lung) efficiency;
★ Improved muscle strength and endurance;
★ Reduced body fat;
★ Increased lean muscle mass;
★ Sharper mental focus and discipline;
★ The ability to work out effectively wherever you are in the minimum amount of time available.

TOTAL FITNESS FOR ALL

I have never yet met a client who hasn't seen considerable results after following the 4-week program – and my clients have been incredibly diverse, ranging from sedentary, overweight businessmen who may start out being unable to run round the block, to professional athletes whose problem might be a psychological block. Two of my better-known clients – Pierce Brosnan and Geri Halliwell – couldn't be more different in terms of body type (obviously!) and their workout goals are different too, but the program has achieved great results in both cases.

When Pierce trained with me, he was looking to reduce his body fat and increase his lean muscle definition – essential for those shirtless scenes that are obligatory when you're playing 007. But his fitness also has to be functional because the role of Bond is extremely physically demanding. When you see him running after a villain in a scene, it really is Pierce doing it – and he has usually done each scene many times in quick succession. It's essential that he has the cardiovascular and muscle strength that will allow him to repeat a physically demanding scene over and over again without looking hot, sweaty and red in the face. Nor could he be out of breath as he may have had lines to deliver.

This level of fitness is reached in the minimum amount of time a day – a movie schedule is run very much like a military operation and the stars have to fit in 30-minute sessions before or after rehearsals and filming.

While Geri Halliwell doesn't yet have to perform any action hero stunts, she does have a schedule that is physically highly demanding. She needs the stamina and muscle strength to complete a 2-hour choreographed live performance or a video shoot that might involve repeating dance routines for 8 hours a day. She has achieved this high level of fitness with the cardiovascular and weight-training techniques described in this book, together with her yoga. One of the highlights for her last year was playing to US and British troops stationed in the desert in Oman. Running on the beach the next day with me and her bodyguard, the troops were impressed at her level of fitness. (And to the women reading this who are worried that a military-style training program will leave them looking masculine and bulked-up, Geri is a living example that training with weights does not bulk you up – it simply tones and forms the physique, ultimately resulting in a smaller overall body shape.)

As I found working on the last two James Bond movies with Denise Richards and, more recently, Halle Berry, acting on a movie set is also very strict and certain looks have to be achieved at the same time as keeping a clear head for all those lines. The Commando Workout is so fast and effective with its 30-minute sessions that it is perfect for movie set workouts. These women maintain a high level of fitness and their action sequences are the result of hard work and dedication.

WHO IS THIS PROGRAM FOR?

★ Anyone who wants to achieve something worthwhile;
★ Anyone with a busy life and not much time to spare who wants to see great results;
★ Anyone who really wants to get into exceptional physical and mental shape;
★ Anyone who wants to break the disappointing cycle of fitness efforts – getting in shape and out of shape and always seeming to end up 'out' rather than 'in'!
★ Anyone who struggles to stay focused and disciplined who would like to get better at reaching their long-term goals;
★ Anyone at a low point in their life, physically or mentally, looking for a new direction;
★ Anyone who enjoys a challenge and the chance to compete against themselves.

GETTING PREPARED FOR ACTION

You may be impatient to get started and tempted to skip straight to Chapter 8 where the 4-week program starts. But one of the most important life-lessons I learned from my military training is that the right preparation can mean the difference between success and failure. This is your first test of discipline!

This program is not an easy option – that is why it works. Without the right preparation, you won't get to the end. But if you read, digest and put into action Chapters 2–7 first, you are giving yourself an almost 100% guaranteed chance of success.

FACT AND FICTION – WISE UP NOW

But before going any further, there are a lot of myths floating around about exercise; they are not helpful and some of them deter beginners from even trying to get fit. So let's set the record straight before we get started:

Fiction: The longer you devote to each workout, the better the results.
Fact: It's the quality not the quantity that counts and the Commando Workout program enables you to build fitness in just 30 minutes a day.

'I just don't have enough time to devote to exercise to get results' is an excuse I hear time and time again for not exercising at all. Many people think that unless you can devote 2 hours a day to the gym it's not worth bothering. However busy you are, you will find a 30-minute slot in your day for a workout if you really want to. (If you can find 30 minutes a day to watch TV, then you can find the same time for exercise.)

The 4-week program is also designed to increase your mental strength, which means that you'll be sharper throughout the day. You may well find that you can complete everyday tasks with more efficiency – the end result being more free time in general!

Fiction: You get the best results working out in a gym with special equipment.
Fact: Gyms may provide a beautiful environment, but there are many ways to build fitness without machines and gimmicks.

I've done a workout in a derelict house in the middle of a war zone in Bosnia. I lived in an igloo for 7 days in Norway and worked out every day on the snow and ice. Commando squadrons based with the Marines spend a lot of time on ships and will work out on the flight deck while the ship is moving up and down.

This book will equip you so you can workout anywhere – at home, at work, in a hotel room. Yes, you can do this workout in a gym, but you'll get just as good results doing it at home and outdoors. It is about using your imagination and the knowledge of fitness that you'll learn from this program – and the fresh air and long summer evenings.

Fiction: After exercising you should feel tired.
Fact: The Commando Workout will increase your stamina and make you feel more awake and alive than ever before.

'I'm just too tired to exercise' is another favourite excuse. If you really feel like you have no energy at the end of the day for exercise, then it is more vital than ever that you start on this program! Although some people do feel more tired during the initial stages of a

workout program, I can guarantee that as you get into it you will notice your energy levels soaring. Technically, this is because the program is going to increase your body's ability to make ATP (adenosine triphosphate), the energy supply used by every cell in the body. That means you're going to wake up with more energy and feel less tired throughout your working day.

Fiction: *If you exercise you can eat what you want.*
Fact: *Commandos eat quite a lot of food, but they are well educated about which foods make the best fuels for a healthy body and are choosy about what they eat.*

When exercising, it is even more important than ever to eat correctly and to give the body exactly what it needs. It is easy to think that if you're doing 6 sessions a week, then you should be able to eat anything and stay slim. Sadly, this is simply not the case. It's very simple – if you put more calories in than you're burning off, then you will gain weight. And there's more to good eating than not overdoing the calories. Food is fuel and without the right fuel you won't get the best out of your exercise sessions. We'll look at exactly what you should be eating in Chapter 3.

Fiction: *Exercising at a moderate level burns more fat.*
Fact: *The chemistry of exercise and fuel consumption is complex but it is important that you don't let statements like this lull you into shying away from the harder sessions in your workouts.*

The exercise industry gave out some misleading information in the 80s and early 90s that some people still believe is true. Namely, that there is a magic 'fat-burning' zone for exercise which involves working at around 60% of your maximum heart rate. The theory was that keeping workouts at this moderate level means your body burns off the maximum amount of fat for energy.

It is true that at a moderate level, the body uses a higher *percentage* of fat for fuel. But it's also true that the body uses the *highest* percentage of fat for fuel when it is completely at rest. And we all know that you don't get slim by lying down! The fact is, when it comes to weight loss it is the *total energy expenditure* that counts.

For example: you do a 20-minute run at a moderate pace and burn around 200 calories. Do the same 20-minute run at the fastest pace you can sustain for this period and you burn 350–400 calories. Now, which activity do you think is going to result in the most weight loss if repeated regularly? That's right – the harder you work, the more calories you expend. It doesn't matter what percentage of these calories are fat. What matters is the *total calorie deficit* you have created. When your body doesn't have enough calories to sustain all its daily activities, it turns to just one source for energy – stored body fat – and that's what we want it to do. Please don't forget this.

Fiction: *The only way to burn calories is to do cardio work.*
Fact: *Resistance training is the key to a long-term efficient metabolism.*

Cardiovascular work (such as walking, running, swimming and cycling) is an essential part of a fat-burning program because it creates a calorie deficit. But weight training is an equally vital part of weight management. Weight training, also known as strength training or resistance training, increases lean muscle tissue. And muscle is what we call 'metabolically active' – it requires a lot of calories for maintenance even in its resting state. So, the more lean muscle tissue you have, the more calories – and body fat – you'll burn off, even when you are asleep.

This is one reason why many people gain weight as they get older – muscle wastage is a natural part of the ageing process. Unless you have a strenuous manual job or do some regular form of strength training, you will lose around ½lb (0.23kg) lean muscle tissue a year – and your metabolic rate will drop accordingly. The program is designed to redress this balance by increasing your lean muscle mass and boosting your metabolic rate.

Fiction: *Working with weights always builds bulky muscles.*
Fact: *Bodybuilders use specific techniques to achieve that bulked-up look and they are not included here.*

The program is designed to develop total body fitness and the pay-off is a lean, defined, balanced body shape. Women in particular (because they don't have enough testosterone for the required muscle growth) will find this program shrinks rather than increases their body size. Weight is not an issue here. I have trained women whose dress sizes went gone down by 2 or 3 sizes but they remained the same weight. It is your shape that counts.

CHAPTER 1: KEY POINTS

★ You don't need to spend hours a day in a gym to get results.

★ You do need to commit to work hard.

★ You'll achieve much more on this program than just weight loss.

★ You'll get results whether you're male or female – and whatever your fitness levels.

★ You'll learn the skills you need to keep yourself in shape for the rest of your life.

MOTIVATION FOR ACTION

If you feel like you're at a low ebb – overweight, unfit, directionless – then congratulations! You are at the ideal place to start this program from. In fact, in the early stages of the commando training program in the forces, the whole military philosophy is to break you down before they build you up. Physical Training Instructors (PTIs) put you through a systemic process designed to break your will so you don't even know who you are anymore. Then they set about building you up, step-by-step, until you are full of the confidence that lets you know for sure that you're the best.

The Commando Workout is not designed to break you down or make you feel bad, but it will build up your confidence in your physical and mental strength so that by the end you will feel just as proud of your achievement as do the candidates who pass the commando course.

YOUR MENTAL WARM-UP

Getting in the right frame of mind before you start is the key to a productive and, yes, *enjoyable* exercise. Warming up the mind is just as important as warming up the body. In some ways, your mind is your most important 'muscle'; if your mind is not in shape you will find it much harder to achieve your goals. When you are in the right frame of mind, you will find you can accomplish a lot more than you expect. That is why commandos train their minds for the mental toughness to take them where they want to go – and that is why this program is going to make a long-term difference.

I can't overemphasize the importance of mental dialogue. Your mind is like a heat-seeking missile – it moves towards the image you create of yourself, be that positive or negative. If your inner dialogue is constantly negative and critical (*'What's the point of doing this exercise?', 'I'm not good enough', 'I'll always be fat'*), your mind will accept these thoughts as reality and shape your behaviour accordingly. So, if you have a mental image of yourself as lazy, uncoordinated and unathletic, then that is how you will act. Think of yourself as overweight and out of shape, and that's what you'll be. But think of yourself as a strong, fit person and you'll start to act like one – and become one! By the same token, stay away from anyone or anything that is negative.

SILENCING THE INNER CRITIC

Have some replies ready for that sabotaging voice in your head. If the negative voice says, *'What's the point of five more repetitions? It hurts and I'll always be fat and useless'*, then tell it to shut up – either in your head or out loud if you want. Replace your negative thoughts with positive statements such as *'I am doing well', 'I am good at this', 'I am getting stronger'* and *'I am enjoying this'* and know that every day you are getting closer to your goal of becoming lean, strong and fit. Yes, you may be out of shape now, but focusing on the negative will only prevent you from seeing and experiencing the positive.

If your inner voice tells you to do one less repetition because you are tired, don't give in. Ignore the voice and you'll feel 200% better when you have finished the job and done your best. If your inner voice tells you to turn off the alarm because missing one session won't make any difference, say, *'Yes it will – the fewer sessions I miss, the quicker I'll see results.'* It is a simple equation, but positive thoughts really do equal positive action and it is all about being disciplined and honest with yourself.

TRAINING YOURSELF TO ENJOY HARD WORK

It is human nature to gravitate towards what's pleasurable rather than painful – but real change demands real work. To a large extent, whether you see exercise as pleasurable or painful depends on your own perception. Think of the 'mental tape' of thoughts that runs through your mind while you work out. Is your tape negative, worrying about the workout or is it positive, urging you on to succeed? You can work a lot harder and achieve considerably better results by giving yourself a positive 'mental tape'.

So, switch off your negative mental tape (*'I'm too tired'*, *'I'm really sweating'*, *'I can't carry on'*, *'My muscles are killing me'*, *'I can't do much more of this'*) and replace it with a positive one (*'This is my favourite track'*, *'This is a beautiful day'*, *'My muscles feel so strong'*, *'I'm really moving now'*, *'I will achieve my goals'*). You'll find that not only are you able to work harder, but exercise feels easier and you feel stronger and more energized. This is not 'psycho babble' – it is attitude training to make sure you get results and keep getting results.

When you get out of bed for your early-morning workout, stop for a moment and listen to what's going through your head. Your natural inclination may be to run a mental tape along the lines of *'I am so tired'*, *'I can't believe I'm doing this'*, *'I must be mad, this is awful'*, *'I wish I was back asleep.'* Are you surprised, then, that when you start your workout it feels like hard work?

It may feel unnatural to begin with, but try repeating a positive dialogue to yourself and see what a difference it makes. Say out loud, *'I'm really up for this workout'*, *'I'm going to give it my best', 'This is a turning point for me', 'This program is a challenge but I know I can do it and it's going to change my life and habits for the better'.*

USING YOUR SENSES

You may have heard athletes talking about 'the zone' – that sought-after mental state where mind and body feel ultimately focused together on achieving their sporting best. One can't work without the other. In the military too, this state of special alertness is valued and encouraged. Each of the senses has an important role to play in how you behave and we can train ourselves to use sound, vision and even the sense of smell to become more effective and motivated people.

SIGHT

How we think we look has a big impact on how we act. Most people will be working out at least in part because they want to feel better about the way they look – and this is nothing to be ashamed of! Having strong visual images of your goals will help you to reach them.

Feeling unhappy with your body shape – whether it is because you can't fit into your clothes, you feel people make judgements about your personality based on the way you look, or because you're not getting the kind of reaction you'd like from the opposite sex – can all have a serious impact on your confidence and self-esteem. Wanting to improve the way you look is a valid and worthwhile goal, but you'll be happier with the results and much more successful in achieving your goal if you define it with a clear vision before you start. If you simply aim to look 'better' or look 'fantastic', how will you know when you've got there? This is where visual tools come in. Here are some suggestions – choose and use whichever works for you:

★ A snapshot of yourself when you looked your best.

★ A pair of jeans you used to fit into or a new pair in a size you'd like to fit into.

★ A picture of a celebrity, model or sports star who you think looks great.

★ A belt set at a notch you used to be able to fasten.

SOUND

Sounds – both in your external workout environment and those made by your body, such as your breathing – all make a difference to effective training. When you are focused on your training you will be aware of your breathing, the regular pounding of your feet and how hard your heart is working. If you have never really noticed these sounds, make a special effort next time you are out for a jog or walk – you'll find that your workout gains a more natural rhythm and that there is an improved inner focus for your training sessions.

There is no disputing that music is a powerful motivator – ask any marketing guru and they'll tell you that the right music will make customers spend more money in the mall, or eat more in a restaurant! Music has the power to evoke emotions, trigger memories and influence your mood. So it is worthwhile taking the time to source the right music for your workout sessions – it can make the difference between pushing yourself to finish the last 5 minutes or ending your session early. A portable CD or cassette player is a worthwhile investment – make sure you buy one that's designed to be used for exercise (that will still play while being jogged about). Tapes or CDs are a better bet than tuning into a radio station – there's nothing more demotivating than reaching the last 5 minutes of your treadmill run when you are really having to dig deep and the station you're listening to switches to the news or a slow, romantic number.

A WORD ON SAFETY

If you're running or cycling outdoors, never listen to music when you are near traffic – for obvious reasons you need to be able to hear approaching cars. If you are exercising outdoors after dark or in a remote area, it is a good idea to be able to hear anyone approaching you.

Do note, however, that music does not work for everyone. Many professional athletes prefer to work out in silence because they are fully tuned into how their body feels and music would detract from this mental focus. You might find that you reach this state of mind towards the end of the 4-week program. Also, if you've had a stressful day at work, working out in silence can offer your brain the oasis of calm it needs to recuperate. If the workout tape that normally gets you up and running is irritating you, then switch it off and carry on without it.

SMELL

Can smell really influence your motivation? You bet it can! Our sense of smell is a powerful, though seldom fully conscious influence on how we act. By becoming aware of our sense of smell we become more attuned to our environment – more alert and more physically alive. In the military, soldiers use their sense of smell to detect the whereabouts of other people. Although you won't be needing this particular skill in your 4-week workout, it is definitely worth your while to pay attention to this undervalued sense – especially while training out of doors.

The use of smell is one of the reasons it's good to do your early morning workout in the open air. You may not feel great when you drag yourself out of bed, but take in a few gulps of fresh, clear morning air and I guarantee you'll start to feel better. When exercising at home, you can experiment with burning essential oils in your workout environment. Studies have shown that the smell of peppermint oil can help exercisers work out for longer.

You'll also probably notice that as you become fitter, your senses become more finely tuned, heightening your senses of smell and taste. Time and time again, I have noticed that after a few weeks of training, a client will voluntarily give up or cut down on smoking. My theory is that as the senses become heightened, you instinctively seek out or create a clean environment to exist in. Cigarettes simply no longer appeal.

TRAINING PARTNERS – GET YOURSELF AN EXERCISE BUDDY

Commandos in the field use what is known as the 'buddy-buddy' system to take care and look out for each other. On a more everyday level, you and your buddy will act as personal motivators for each other. Got to go for a run? Then your buddy will be knocking on your door to ensure you make it. About to set off on a 2-day cross-country hike? Your buddy will check that your kit is intact before you go. And you do the same for him.

If you have a friend who also wants to get in great shape, why don't you suggest they join you on the 4-week program as your buddy? Choose your buddy carefully and make a pact to encourage and motivate each other along the way. So, when one of you says, 'I'm tired, I don't think I can make our session tonight,' the other will be there to talk you round and insist you come along. Getting out of bed and outdoors at 6.30am can be tough at times, but it will definitely be easier if you know there is a buddy waiting in the park to run or walk with you. Knowing that you will be letting a friend down as well as yourself by missing a session is usually enough for most people to ensure they turn up!

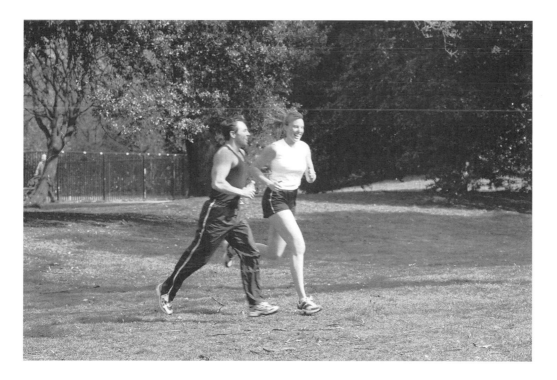

PREPARATION

One of the most enduring lessons the military teaches is that there are several practical steps you can take to aid your motivation. One of the most important is preparation.

As a commando, you are on 24-hour notice to respond to any crisis anywhere in the world. What makes this logistical feat possible is intelligent and thorough preparation. In day-to-day life, the right preparation will also make the difference between reaching, or missing, your personal goals.

People assume that motivation is 'all in the mind' – that it's a purely psychological process. It is true that drive and commitment do come from the mind, but mental focus does not arrive by magic. If you wait until the motivation to exercise arrives, you will wait for a very long time! Put in the mental and practical forward planning before your workouts and it will be a lot easier to get started when the time comes.

When you begin this program, your mind is likely to be looking for obstacles that it can use as an excuse not to work out. Small obstacles such as *'The alarm didn't go off'* or *'I couldn't find my trainers'* can have a big effect when doing something new, so you will need to find ways to ensure that such obstacles do not get between you and your work-out. By careful forward planning – anticipating and removing the setbacks before you meet them – you will remove these predictable obstacles and gain the upper hand.

Early morning exercise sessions require the following checklist before you go to bed:

★ Is your kit clean and laid out next to your bed ready for you to jump into it when you get up?
★ Are your running shoes ready?
★ If you are exercising at home, is your exercise space clear of clutter?
★ Have you set your alarm clock to wake you in good time?
★ Are your work clothes ready for you to get into after your workout and shower so you are not late for work?
★ Do you have the ingredients for breakfast in the fridge so you can replenish your energy stores before you go to work?

★ Have you checked the 30-day program and mentally gone through the next day's session so you don't waste time in the morning figuring out what you need to do?

You also need to be thinking ahead to your second workout session later in the day. The night before, have a look at what's involved and decide where you are going to do it. If you are planning to do it after work, it is a good idea to pick a venue (perhaps a gym or park) near to your workplace, so that it is easy for you to travel immediately from work into your exercise session. Simply think of that extra 30–45 minute session as an extension to the working day. Alternatively, if you have enough time to do your workout at lunchtime, you'll have the satisfaction of knowing you can go home and relax at the end of the day.

Make sure you do *go home and relax*, not join your colleagues in the nearest bar. A few beers after work to wind down might not seem like the biggest vice in the world, but if you do so regularly, you'll be consuming a substantial quantity of nutrient-bankrupt calories while draining your body of vital vitamins and minerals. As well as this, forcing your body to use energy to process alcohol means that there is less energy available to fuel your muscles and cardiovascular system when you come to do your next workout.

For your lunchtime/evening session your checklist requires the following:

★ Have you packed your bag with the kit for your second daily workout to take with you to work if you're doing your session at lunchtime or straight after work? (Have a second set of clean clothes in your bag, a second water bottle and towel, so all you need to do is add your trainers after your morning session and then you're ready to go).
★ Have you planned the venue for your second session and mentally gone through what's involved?
★ Have you got the ingredients at home for your evening meal to replenish your energy stores after your workout?

KEEPING YOUR DAILY WORKOUT RECORD

With each day of your 30-day program there is a box in which to record that day's exercise achievements. Keeping a log of your workout sessions allows you to track your progress – to look back and see how far you've come. When you're engrossed in an exercise program, you can go through phases when you feel like you're not getting anywhere. Comparing today's workout with what you were doing 10 days ago is a quick and indisputable way of reminding yourself that you are progressing. It also allows you to see where you've been going wrong if you are not getting the results you want. Are you completing most workouts? Are you working at the right intensity? You'll find the answer by looking back at your daily training log.

Here is an example of a training log and how to fill it out:

GOAL	COMPLETED
30 min powerwalk/jog	20 mins walking/10 mins jogging
Press-ups 5–8–15–8–5	5–8–10–6–5
Bentover row 5–8–15–8–5	5–8–15–8–5
Shoulder press 5–8–15–8–5	5–8–15–8–5
Bicep curls 5–8–15–8–5	5–8–15–8–5
Tricep dips 5–8–15–8–5	5–8–9–8–5
Effort level	9
Energy	7–8
Enjoyment	9
Overall performance	7–8

COMMENTS:
Unable to complete the full number of press-ups and tricep dips but overall a good session. Did ab workout after cardio session. Felt full of energy all day after the AM workout but was a little tired during PM workout. Missed afternoon snack – could this be why?

CHAPTER 2: KEY POINTS

★   The more planning and preparation you put into your workouts, the more likely you are to complete them.

★   Getting in the right frame of mind before you start is the key to enjoying your exercise session.

★   Your senses can be powerful motivational tools, if you know how to use them.

★   Keep a detailed log of the training you've completed to track your progress.

★   Don't go it alone – working with a buddy can keep you on track.

FUEL FOR FITNESS:

THE COMMANDO POWER EATING PLAN

There's an old saying that an army marches on its stomach and it's true that without plenty of adequate fuel from food, there's no way anyone could keep up with the pace demanded by the military. The idea of a commando going on a diet sounds crazy – their lifestyle demands powerful nutritional fuel.

But many of you reading this will be motivated to follow the program because you feel you are overweight. So this leaves a dilemma – how to be sure you are eating a large enough amount of food to fuel an intensive physical program without getting run down, but still lose the excess weight. It sounds impossible, but it is not, nor does it involve complicated diet plans. The first thing to understand is that 'diets' don't work. Diets, or restrictive eating plans, whether the low-carbohydrate diet, the grapefruit diet or the cabbage soup diet, do not see food as a 'friend' – as the valuable fuel that it is. Instead, they see food as the 'enemy' – as something largely to be avoided – and such diets are not viable long-term solutions to weight management. Although you may lose weight quickly at first, it is not fat you are losing, but water and muscle. And as muscle is more metabolically active than fat, the immediate result is that your metabolic rate is lowered. So, after your initial weight loss, you will inevitably find that you put on weight because your body is using up fewer calories. If you take your health, strength and fitness seriously, you will not follow a restricted diet of this sort.

The other extreme – eating however much or whatever you want – is just as disastrous. It is tempting to think that if you are doing several intensive exercise sessions a week, then you can eat as much as you like and still stay in great shape. Not true. After all, it doesn't take a rocket scientist to work out that if you burn off 350 calories during your exercise session, but reward yourself with a pizza and a couple of beers which clock in at 1,500 calories, you're not going to achieve that lean, sculpted shape of your dreams anytime soon.

It is very simple – if you put more calories in than you're putting out, then you will start gaining weight. Your calorie allowance is like a budget – if you overspend you will get into debt (put on fat).

Also, regular exercise is not a get-out clause from paying attention to the food you eat. Like a motor engine, our body works more efficiently if we give it high quality fuel. Feeding our bodies with high calorie foods with little nutritional worth can only lead to disaster in the long term and you will find that you cannot perform to the best of your abilities.

This means eating enough carbohydrate to restock your energy stores after cardiovascular activities such as running. It also means eating enough protein so that your muscles can repair themselves and grow stronger after every Power Circuit. And it means ensuring you eat enough fresh produce to provide the essential minerals and vitamins for optimum health – including your vital immune defences.

The Commando Power Eating Plan is based on the KIS principle – Keep It Simple. The key is eating the right foods at the right time of day to balance your blood glucose levels so that you feel consistently energetic and avoid energy slumps. The plan involves eating 5 times a day, but in smaller amounts than you would normally on a traditional 3-meal-a-day diet. Eating little and often means you will never feel hungry. You will always have the required energy to do a good workout and you will also avoid the dreaded post-lunch lethargy. Fact – every time you eat you raise your metabolism by 10–15%.

Ever wondered what the phrase 'you are what you eat' really means? Every cell in your body is constantly being regenerated and your skin, brain, muscle, bone and blood cells all come from the same source – food. So, the better the quality of the food you're eating, the better body you're able to build. Eating processed food has the opposite effect – it actually depletes the body of nutrients as it processes the artificial flavours, preservatives and additives. By eating well, you'll not only feel better on a day-to-day basis, but you'll also look healthier and more vital.

THE COMMANDO POWER EATING PLAN

The Commando Power Eating Plan is based on sound nutritional principles and is designed to get your body in the best possible shape during the 4-week program. You will not go hungry at any stage and you will not be required to eat any foods that you dislike – but there are 8 rules that should be followed.

RULE 1 – DO NOT SKIP MEALS.

A commando would never miss a meal as without the dietary fuel they run the risk of being ineffective to themselves and to their colleagues. Going hungry will disrupt your steady blood sugar levels and can affect your mood as well as energy levels. You will need to be disciplined about your eating habits – making sure you eat the right amounts at the right times – if you are to make a success of this program.

RULE 2 – NO FOOD TO BE CONSUMED BEFORE YOUR MORNING PYRAMID POWERWALK/JOG.

Breakfast should wait until after your workout. Doing your morning workout on an empty stomach means that your body is forced to draw on fat reserves for fuel. If you eat before your workout, your body will use this food for fuel instead. And doing your Pyramid Powerwalk/Jog first thing in the morning kick-starts your metabolic rate so you will burn more calories throughout the rest of the day.

RULE 3 – EAT A CARBOHYDRATE-BASED BREAKFAST AFTER YOUR PYRAMID POWERWALK/JOG.

It is important to refuel as soon as possible after exercise, as the production and storage of glycogen (muscle fuel) is fastest during the 2 hours immediately following a workout and this will ensure you have enough fuel for your evening workout.

RULE 4 – EAT A MIXED PROTEIN/CARBOHYDRATE SNACK MID-MORNING.

The most efficient way to refuel glycogen is to eat small amounts of complex carbohydrate throughout the day. By eating protein at the same time, you will slow down the rate at which the carbohydrate is absorbed, preventing a fast blood sugar rise. This guarantees a slow, sustained energy release rather than a fast sugar rush, followed by a dip. Plus, every time you eat, you raise your metabolic rate by 20% for around 1 hour afterwards, so eating little and often will keep it revved up throughout the day.

RULE 5 – HAVE A MIXED PROTEIN/CARBOHYDRATE LUNCH.

Studies have shown that the protein needs of strength trainers are greater than those of sedentary people, to compensate for increased protein breakdown in the muscles during training and to promote new growth and tissue repair. However, contrary to popular belief, protein above the body's requirements is not converted into muscle tissue.

Eating a mix of carbohydrate and protein at lunch helps you avoid the post-lunch energy slump – again, you'll experience a slow, sustained rise in blood sugar rather than a fast peak followed by a dip.

RULE 6 – HAVE A CARBOHYDRATE SNACK 1–2 TWO HOURS BEFORE YOUR POWER CIRCUIT.

Because carbohydrate, in the form of blood glucose and muscle glycogen, is the main fuel used during strength training, it is crucial that you optimise your carbohydrate stores prior to your evening Power Circuit workout.

RULE 7 – HAVE AN EVENING MEAL AFTER YOUR POWER CIRCUIT WORKOUT OF PROTEIN AND VEGETABLES.

Restricting your starchy carbohydrate intake in the evenings will ensure that you don't take in excess calories at the time of day when your body is at rest and likely to store them as fat. It also means that you are more likely to base your meals around vegetables, ensuring you get your daily quota. Restricting your carbohydrate at this point also leaves your glycogen levels depleted so that your body is forced to draw on fat reserves to fuel the morning workout.

RULE 8 – DRINK AT LEAST 2 LITRES (3½ PINTS) OF STILL WATER A DAY.

The human body is 75% water. You can survive for days without food but just a 2% loss of the water surrounding your cells will mean a 20% fall in your energy levels – as well as affecting the condition of your skin and your ability to concentrate. The standard advice is to drink 8 large glasses a day but you may need twice this amount if you are exercising regularly. The easiest way to tell if you are drinking enough is by the colour of your urine – it should be a light straw colour. The darker it is, the more you need to drink. And as for whether to drink bottled or tap water, did you know that tap water has to undergo 57 tests for possible contaminants, and bottled water only 15? And tap water is free! If you don't like the taste of your local water, invest in a water filter (around £20 from department stores) – it does improve the taste.

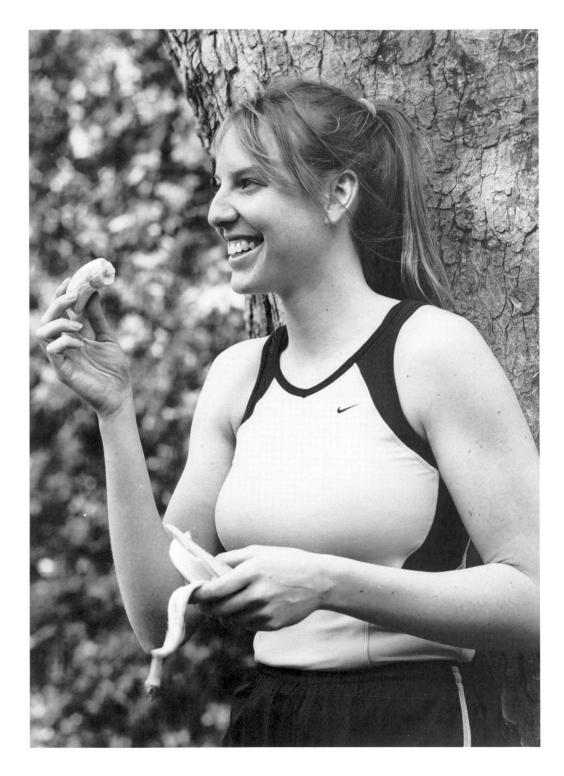

CHOOSING WHAT TO EAT

Once again, Keep It Simple comes in to play:

★ Buy in advance and plan your meals so you don't end up grabbing at convenience food or take-outs because you are out of fresh produce.
★ Prepare food as simply as possibly – grill chicken and fish, serve vegetables steamed, boiled or grated raw. Avoid adding fat or sauces – use spices and fresh herbs for extra flavour.
★ Think in portions. One portion equals the size of your clenched fist.
★ Think about how a food will make you feel as you're eating it, immediately after you've eaten it and an hour after you've eaten it. If you know it will make you feel bloated, overweight or guilty, then go for something that won't!
★ Eat as few ready-made, processed meals as possible.
★ Buy the best quality food you can afford – fresh fruit and vegetables and meat whenever possible.
★ Don't let food control you – you control food and you have the power.

SOME MEAL SUGGESTIONS

Breakfasts

Wholegrain toast with 1 poached egg and a glass orange juice
Porridge made with skimmed milk and half a sliced banana
Banana and strawberry smoothie made with natural yoghurt and a splash of milk
Omelette made with the whites of 3 eggs and one slice of toast.

Mid-morning snacks

Handful of nuts or seeds
Low-fat yoghurt and chopped fresh fruit
Apple and small piece of cheese
Berry smoothie (made with natural yoghurt)
Metrx (protein supplement) – ½ sachet or 1 bar.

Lunches

Turkey/ham/lean beef with grated vegetable salad

Jacket potato with low-fat cottage cheese or tuna and sweet corn

Grilled salmon with brown rice salad and fresh tomatoes

Pasta salad with lentils and lots of salad greens.

Afternoon snacks

Rice cakes with low-fat spread or low-sugar jam

Slice of rye bread and cottage cheese

Fresh fruit salad and natural yoghurt

No sugar, low fat cereal bar or ½ sachet Metrx.

Evening meals

Choose a main meal protein, cooked without fat:

chicken breast	shellfish (such as crab,
turkey breast	prawns)
lean ham	eggs (just the whites)
lean minced beef	cottage cheese
sirloin steak	beans
fish (such as cod, haddock,	lentils
salmon, sea bass, swordfish, tuna)	tofu

Serve with a portion of:

broccoli	lettuce
carrots	beetroot
courgettes	asparagus
spinach	Brussels sprouts
cabbage	onions
tomatoes	leek
squash	

GOOD FATS/BAD FATS

You've probably read a lot about the importance of eating a low-fat diet to cut back on excess weight and reduce the risk of heart disease. But cutting fat completely out of the diet is not the answer. A diet containing no fats whatsoever is actually bad for your health and some fats are essential to keep your body in good working order. We tend to think of fats only in terms of their calorific value – as no more than a fuel. But research has proved that fat is not only a valuable source of energy, but the right fats will also protect you against illness and are vital for the production and distribution of the hormones testosterone, oestrogen and progesterone around the body. There are 2 main types of fat – saturated and unsaturated.

Saturated fats

These are generally considered 'bad' fats. They are solid at room temperature and tend to come from animal products such as butter, margarine, lard, suet, meat, eggs, milk, cheese and yoghurt. Cakes, biscuits and pastry – including pasties and pie crusts, which are generally made from margarine or butter – are likely to be high in saturated fats. Foods such as these should form only a very limited part of your diet. Too much saturated fat and you will increase your risk of heart disease and other long-term health problems.

Unsaturated fats

Otherwise known as mono- and polyunsaturated fats, these tend to be liquid at room temperature. The key healthy fats are in this group and it is essential that your diet contains them. Typically, they come from vegetable sources, namely oils such as olive, sunflower, safflower, rapeseed, soya, peanut and sesame. They are also found in soft margarines labelled 'high in polyunsaturates'.

Of particular importance are two key polyunsaturates – omega-3 and omega-6 essential fatty acids (EFAs). These are found in oily fish such as salmon, anchovies, mackerel, herring, trout, mullet and sardines, and have been shown to help prevent heart disease and some types of cancer. They also have been shown to improve skin health.

Improving your dietary fat profile

The problem is that most of us eat too much fat and often the wrong type of fat. You can get enough simply by eating oily fish twice a week, and using 1 tablespoon of oil in cooking or dressings every day.

EASY WAYS TO LIMIT YOUR FAT INTAKE

1 Grill, steam or microwave food without adding any fat.
2 If frying, use a non-stick pan and add a minimal amount of oil.
3 Choose lean meats and trim off any visible fat before cooking.
4 Avoid sausages, salami, patés and pies.
5 Opt for low-fat yoghurt, cheese, and skimmed milk.

THE DOS AND DON'TS OF EATING WELL

1 **Do eat little and often.**
2 **Do eat slowly. It gives your stomach time to send signals to your brain to say that it is full and it also helps you digest food efficiently. Chew your food properly before you swallow – put your knife and fork down between mouthfuls.**
3 **Do drink plenty of water throughout the day but avoid drinking more than 1 glass with a meal – it can dilute your digestive enzymes.**
4 **Don't eat on the couch in front of the TV. The couch will make you slump, leading to bad digestion. Instead, sit in a comfortable position at a table.**
5 **Don't drink alcohol with your meals – your body will use the alcohol for energy and store the food calories as fat.**
6 **Do limit the amount of foods in your diet that contain a lot of sugar.**
7 **And finally, if you are still hungry at the end of your meal, do bear in mind that it takes 10 minutes for your body's chemical messengers to tell your brain that you are full up. Try waiting 10 minutes to see if you really are still hungry for more.**

ABOUT PROTEIN DRINKS

Many gyms sell supplements and drinks that are claimed to help you reach your training goals. In particular, protein-based drinks are marketed as aids to increasing muscle mass and strength and this might seem appealing if you feel you're too skinny.

Most protein drinks are based around powdered milk and/or egg protein (soya is also available), and may contain a source of carbohydrate such as glucose polymers, as well as amino acids, vitamins and minerals.

Taking a protein-based supplement can contribute to your daily protein intake but will not encourage muscle growth at a faster rate than protein from a food source. They can, however, be a convenient substitute for your daily mid-morning or afternoon snack if you are pressed for time. Choose a brand, such as Metrx, that is low in fat and sugar and that comes in sachets. Mix ½ sachet with water and ice for a snack.

Remember, extra protein over and above your requirements is not turned into muscle!

FIVE USEFUL SUPPLEMENTS

A balanced diet will provide your body with all the nutrients it needs. But sometimes it can benefit from a little extra help. Here are 5 supplements that can make a difference.

Probiotics

Probiotics can help with digestion and immune system problems. The body relies on 'friendly' bacteria to help fight off disease, digest food and absorb nutrients. Taking antibiotics can deplete your natural supply of these bacteria, as can stress and poor nutrition. If you suffer from poor digestion or irritable bowel syndrome (IBS), it is worth taking a probiotic – a supplement of 'friendly' bacteria.

Q10 and Carnitine

Q10 and carnitine can improve your body's energy efficiency. Coenzyme Q10, to give it its proper name, is a substance found naturally in every cell in your body. It plays a role in the production of energy and works as an antioxidant protecting the body from the damaging effects of free radicals. Taken in supplement form, it works wonders in boosting energy levels, but it works even better when taken with carnitine. Carnitine is an amino acid naturally produced by the body in the brain, heart and kidneys. It transports fatty acids into the mitochondria (the body's 'power cells').

B vitamins

B-complex vitamins may need a top up if you train regularly. B vitamins are essential for converting food into energy, as well as keeping the nervous system and brain healthy, but they can be depleted by intense exercise. If you're not used to exercising regularly, it could be worth taking a supplement containing all the B vitamins.

Natural help with cravings

If you are finding it difficult to cut down your alcohol intake, try Kudzo, a herbal supplement derived from the root of a Japanese vine that contains a chemical compound, diadzin, that has been found to be effective in curbing cravings for alcohol. To reinforce the benefits of Kudzo, take Milk Thistle, a herbal supplement that encourages liver detoxification. If you are craving chocolate, try eating grapes or a very small amount of a high cocoa chocolate instead.

Glucosamine

Glucosamine helps protect your joints. For years, athletes have taken supplements of glucosamine sulphate – a basic building block in cartilage tissue – to protect against pressure on their joints, especially their knees. Glucosamine is a natural substance found in the human body that helps create connective molecules that form links between cells and tissue. Joint problems are also quite common in the military due to the sheer volume of impact the knees, hips and ankles have to take during training and in action. The Commando Workout is designed for minimum impact on the joints, but if you have suffered from joint problems in the past, you may benefit from a daily dose of 1,500mg of glucosamine before and during the program.

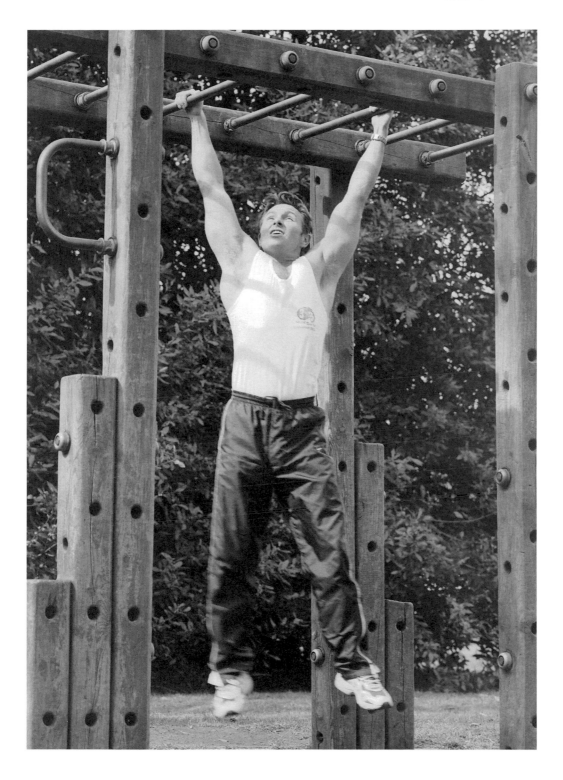

KEEPING A FOOD LOG

On each day of your 30-day program, you need to keep a log of exactly what you have eaten that day. Most nutritionists recommend keeping a food diary when you're trying to improve your eating habits, simply because what we think we've eaten in a day is often a different story from what we've really eaten. Keeping a record of what you have consumed can be useful if you're not getting the results you want. Here's an example of how to fill it out:

FOOD LOG	
FOOD EATEN	**TIME EATEN**
Bowl of porridge with skimmed milk. Banana. Small glass orange juice. Decaf coffee.	8.30am/after morning Powerwalk
Low-fat vanilla yoghurt/large apple. Decaf coffee.	11am
Chicken breast with brown rice and tomato salad/fruit salad.	1.30pm
Protein drink.	4pm
3 slices of ham and mushroom pizza/one small beer.	8.30pm/after evening Power Circuit
Estimated water consumption	3 pints

COMMENTS:
A good day until the evening – didn't have any food at home so relied on take-out. Must go shopping after work tomorrow.

CHAPTER 3: KEY POINTS

★ Food is fuel – give your body the best and you'll achieve the best results.

★ A portion is the size of your fist.

★ Base your eating plan on carbohydrates and protein eaten at specific times of the day.

★ Never eat before your morning training session.

★ Drink at least 2 litres of water a day.

★ Plan and shop for your meals in advance – don't rely on getting the right foods from a restaurant or take-out.

IMPROVISE, ADAPT AND OVERCOME

There is a much-used phrase in the military that sums up the commando philosophy to life – improvise, adapt and overcome. It means dealing with whatever circumstances you find yourself in and using them to your advantage, overcoming physical and mental obstacles and adapting to your environment. It is these principles that are going to make sure you don't miss a single day of your 4-week program!

The program is planned to be followed in the order set out in the book. If this impossible for you, then you can switch around days to suit your schedule – for instance, if you really don't have time to work out one day, then make it the rest day for the week and work out on the day designated as a rest day instead.

But don't think you'll be racing ahead on the program if you miss out the rest days altogether. These are just as important as the exercise sessions. Contrary to popular belief, it is not during an exercise session that your body makes improvements such as increased muscle strength and heart and lung efficiency – it is in the recovery periods afterwards. This is when your body makes 'adaptations' to the stress placed on it during your exercise sessions. Without at least one full day of rest a week, your body will not have the time it needs to recover and adapt fully – you would be bombarding your body with stress until you wear it down and it starts to degenerate, rather than improving your fitness.

MAKE A PLAN AND STICK TO IT

It is a good idea to write your training plans in your diary ahead of the workout. This way your plans will be clear, and you will find it easier to prepare once you have mentally planned ahead by setting your plans out on paper. Sticking to the plan is the simplest, and most effective way to reach your goals.

GOING AWOL – WHAT TO DO IF YOU MISS TRAINING DAYS

Do not try to make up today for what you didn't do yesterday. To succeed at this program you need to rethink your attitude to failure. Don't overdramatise it or use it as an excuse to give up. If you have missed a day's workout, don't try to catch up by doing a double workout the next day – and don't spend the week agonising. Tomorrow is another day – look forward to what you can achieve.

Fill out your training diary for the day you missed with the reason you didn't work out – feeling the effects of a big night out? Deadline at work? Then add a practical solution for avoiding the same scenario cropping up again – say 'no' to that drinks session with your friends; try to delegate some of your workload.

Your program includes two 'AWOL cards' for you to use when you really can't avoid missing a workout. But once these are used up, then missing further sessions will mean you don't get the best from the program. If you have an illness or injury that means you have to miss several days, consider postponing the program until you are back to full health and starting again from the beginning. Remember, you'll only get the best results when you complete all 4 weeks.

WHEN NOT TO TRAIN

You'll do more harm than good and risk a long-term setback if you continue with the program while:

★ **Suffering from a heavy cold or flu.** Do the 'neck check' – if your symptoms are below the neck – aching muscles, coughing, nausea or wheezing – take the day off. If you have a cold with symptoms that are only above the neck – runny nose, sore throat and headache – it's OK to exercise if you feel up to it. Try a 10-minute 'test drive' at half speed. If you feel better after 10 minutes, increase your pace and finish your workout.

★ **Suffering from any illness that means you're not well enough to go to work.**

★ **Suffering from joint pain.** You won't 'exercise through it', but simply make it worse. If you experience knee, shin, ankle or back pain during a workout, see a physiotherapist for advice before you carry on. Get into the habit of listening to your body. One of the keys to avoiding injury is to follow the technique tips for each exercise carefully. In particular avoiding 'locking out' your joints – keep knees and elbows slightly soft (bent) and never rigidly extended. This puts pressure on your joints instead of working your muscles. (See below for more information on exercise injuries.)

★ **Suffering some or all of the symptoms of overtraining.** If you are very keen to succeed it is tempting to do too much too soon. While it is great to have enthusiasm, if you begin to feel any of the following symptoms you may be working too hard and not allowing your body the time it needs to rest and adapt:

  ☆ change of mood and lack of concentration
  ☆ lack of enjoyment in exercise
  ☆ frequent head colds

☆ sleep disturbances

☆ lingering fatigue after exercise sessions

☆ generalised body aches and pains.

For a more accurate diagnosis – one used by athletes – take your pulse first thing in the morning. If it is 10–20 per cent higher than your normal resting heart rate, you need to take at least a day off from training.

NO EXCUSE – JUST DO IT!

The following are NOT excuses to miss a workout:

★ **A hangover.** Just make sure you drink lots of fluid before, during and after your workout as you will be dehydrated.

★ **DOMS – Delayed Onset Muscle Soreness** (that ache you get the day after a good workout). Your 30-day program is designed to take this into account and rest days for muscles are built-in – that's why you always alternate upper and lower body workouts.

★ **Menstruation.** You may feel like you can't work out at that time of the month but many women say that exercise relieves the symptoms of problem periods.

COMMON EXERCISE INJURIES

The program is designed to strengthen your body and prevent exercise injuries. If followed correctly and with good technique, it is very unlikely that you'll get hurt. But it pays to be aware of the signs of an exercise injury. The following injury descriptions and self-treatment advice are not a substitute for the advice of your physician. Always consult a physician or physiotherapist if you experience any of the following:

MUSCLE STRAIN

Area affected: any muscle group.
Symptoms: tenderness, swelling, decreased range of movement.

Cause: damage to muscle tissue.

Treatment: RICE – Rest, Ice, Compression and Elevation of affected area.

STRESS FRACTURE

Area affected: usually in lower leg or foot.

Symptoms: tenderness and swelling.

Cause: sudden increase in the intensity of impact activities like running.

Treatment: rest.

TENDONITIS

Area affected: any tendon, but common in heel of foot (Achilles tendon).

Symptoms: pain, inflammation, restricted movement.

Cause: excessive friction and repetitive strain.

Treatment: ice and ultrasound to reduce inflammation in the short term and rest in the long term.

SHIN SPLINTS

Area affected: front of lower legs.

Symptoms: sharp pain while exercising and walking, sometimes intermittent.

Cause: sudden increase in intensity in training (such as frequent hill running or steps).

Treatment: RICE (as above), then rest and possibly orthotic inserts (*see* page 51) for your running shoes.

ITB SYNDROME (ILIOTIBIAL BAND SYNDROME)

Area affected: outside of thigh from top of hip to knee.

Symptoms: inflammation and soreness during and after activity.

Cause: body imbalances such as flat feet, which throw the knees out of alignment, causing the ITB to rub against the joints of your hip or knee.

Treatment: muscle strengthening exercises and/or orthotic insoles in trainers.

KNEE PAIN

Area affected: front, side, below or behind kneecap.

Symptoms: pain on impact (when walking, climbing stairs, running, etc); swelling.

Cause: muscular imbalances in the legs placing inappropriate pressure on the knee joint.

Treatment: rest, exercises to give joint stability to strengthen legs, orthotics.

SHOULDER PAIN

Area affected: shoulder muscle.

Symptoms: pain when moving arm, restricted range of movement and power in arm.

Cause: overuse or trauma to the rotator cuff (the 4 shoulder muscles).

Treatment: rest and then exercises to strengthen the muscles.

CHAPTER 4: KEY POINTS

★ Don't overtrain.
★ The body is very complex. Get to know it and listen to it.
★ Never be hard on yourself.
★ Always maintain a positive outlook – no matter what!

BEFORE YOU START

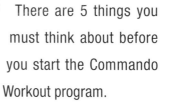

There are 5 things you must think about before you start the Commando Workout program.

1 PICK A 4-WEEK WINDOW THAT IS GOING TO WORK FOR YOU

For best results, you need to follow the 4-week program without missing out any days. It is an intensive program requiring your full commitment. Soldiers' lives are largely planned for them and they have far fewer day-to-day life choices than you. To give yourself the best possible chance of making the program work to your advantage, give some thought as to when you intend to do it. Ideally, you should make a 4-week window when it can be your number one priority (taking into account your responsibilities to your home life and work).

Some life events take a lot of energy and you must be careful not to overcommit yourself. The worst time to do this program is when you have another big commitment such as moving house or changing job. On a smaller scale, it's a good idea to avoid times where you are likely to have a lot of family commitments. (Although sometimes, there's never a right time – if you really want to do it, just go for it!)

Once you've chosen your ideal 4 weeks, record your commitment in your diary and start to plan your life around it. It is only 4 weeks out of your life so you should be able to turn down major social engagements for that duration. As well as putting some of the energy you would normally spend socialising into your workouts, you'll get the best results if you avoid alcohol during the program.

Sometimes, a break from life's basic routine can have a really positive effect on our state of mind. New possibilities become clear and this fresh perspective, combined with the confidence you gain from following the Commando Workout, can bring unexpected benefits as well as renewed physical strength and fitness. You will need to do some planning so, when D-Day comes, there's nothing to stop you getting off to a flying start.

2 CHECK YOUR HEALTH

The most important thing to do before you start is to check that you are in ideal physical shape to complete the program safely. See your doctor before you start this exercise program if:

★ You are overweight. Exercising when overweight can put strain on your heart. Your doctor can check if you have any heart problems that could be made worse by exercise. To check if you're in the healthy weight range, calculate your Body Mass Index, as follows:

☆ Measure your height in metres.
☆ Multiply this figure by itself (for example, 1.7m × 1.7m). This gives your height squared.
☆ Then, measure your weight in kilograms.
☆ Divide your weight by your height squared. This gives you your Body Mass Index.

Healthy	20–24
Overweight	25–29
Obese	30 and above

Some doctors now prefer to measure the waist-to-hip ratio (WHR), because it is thought that fat stored around the abdomen increases the risk of heart problems and other diseases. To calculate your WHR:

☆ Measure your waist at your navel and the hips at the widest point of your bottom.
☆ Divide the waist by the hip measurement. (If your waist measures 32 inches and your hips 37 inches, your WHR is 32 ÷ 37 = 0.86.

	Men	Women
Overweight	0.95 and above	0.86 and above
Average	0.81–0.94	0.71–0.85
Good	below 0.8	below 0.7

★ You have high blood pressure. Hypertension (high blood pressure) is the biggest cause of stroke or heart disease, but it usually shows no symptoms. A normal blood pressure reading is below 130/85, and the ideal is below 120/80. A reading of 140/90 and above means your blood pressure is raised. While regular exercise is an effective way of lowering blood pressure, it is essential that you do it with medical supervision.

★ You have an irregular heartbeat. Heart disease is the world's number one biggest killer and exercise is the best way to reduce your chances of getting it. But an intense exercise program can be dangerous if you already have signs of the disease. You don't need to book in for an ECG (electrocardiogram) to check out your heart – simply pay attention to what it is like after physical exertion such as climbing stairs. See your doctor if your heartbeat is irregular or if it takes a long time to return to normal. And never ignore pains in the chest. They can be a sign of angina – you are not about to have a heart attack, but it does mean there is a problem.

WHEN TO SEE A PHYSIO

Have you ever started on a new fitness regime full of enthusiasm, only to give up a few weeks later because you pick up a niggling knee injury or back strain? At this point, you'd be forgiven for thinking that exercise isn't good for you, and giving up. Although many people don't realise they have a problem until they start exercising, the actual injury is likely to be an accumulation of years of poor posture (from hours spent slumped in front of a computer or steering wheel) and old sports injuries (even from as far back as school).

One solution is to get checked out *before* you start exercising, rather than waiting for an injury to happen. You don't wait to visit the dentist until something goes wrong, so why should you wait for an injury to happen before you visit a physiotherapist?

A large proportion of injuries result from imbalances in muscle strength and flexibility. Subtle imbalances can result in slight changes in the alignment of your joints. Exercising with these changes can significantly increase the stress on the affected joints and muscles. Sometimes it is only a matter of time before 'something goes'. Most people with muscle imbalances have no idea they are there until this happens.

A chartered physiotherapist will prescribe rehabilitation exercises to rebalance any weaknesses and suggest adaptations to your workout to prevent potential problems. Sometimes, all you need is to wear special inserts, called 'orthotics', in your training shoes and these can compensate for flat feet – a common cause of knee pain.

3 CHECK YOU HAVE THE RIGHT KIT AND EQUIPMENT

The Commando Workout program is designed to require the minimum of equipment and expense. But there are some essentials that you need to have in place before you can get started.

TRAINING SHOES

Your most essential piece of equipment is a good cross-trainer (a sports shoe designed both to protect against impact and to keep your foot stable during movement). A good pair of trainers will give you added protection against injury and is a must if you are running. Do not exercise in the trainers you use for everyday wear – instead keep a pair just for your workouts so you get the maximum protection when you need it (wearing them every day soon wears them down). Similarly, if you've had the same pair of training shoes for years, this is an ideal time to invest in a new pair.

If possible, invest in two pairs of training shoes – one for your cardiovascular workouts and one for strength training. Ideally, you should wear a running shoe for your morning cardio sessions – especially if you have had previous knee or ankle problems. When buying your running shoes, try to find a specialist shop where the assistants can give you expert advice on the type of shoes you need. Don't hesitate to ask questions about your shoes – it's important that you get the right pair. A good assistant will take into account your weight and height and ask you what type of ground you will be mainly running on (tarmac, grass, dirt tracks, treadmill, etc) before recommending a shoe.

Failing this, there are some pointers you can use yourself to help you find the right shoe.

★ Try on running shoes towards the end of the day when your feet have swelled to their biggest size. You don't want shoes that fit like a glove – your feet will swell when you run and you want a pair in a size that will allow for this.

★ It may sound obvious, but try on both shoes, lace them up and walk around the shop in them. Check that you can't feel any rubbing from stitching.

★ Look for a shoe that has plenty of material in the sole unit to provide good cushioning and flexibility. If you will be doing your cardio work mainly on a hard surface, look for shoes made especially for road running – they will have longer-wearing soles with extra cushioning for the harder surface. Pay particular attention to the depth of material on the heel of the shoe. This is the part that strikes the ground first with every footfall and it needs to offer enough cushioning to absorb the shock of most of the body's weight landing on a hard surface.

CLOTHING FOR WORKOUTS

Work out in clothes that allow you freedom of movement, and that allow your body to maintain a comfortable temperature. People tend to overdress for outdoor workouts – as a rule of thumb, if you are perfectly warm when you step outside, you will be too hot when you get into your workout. To avoid this problem, dress in layers that can be taken off and stored in a lightweight backpack or tied around your waist when you get warm.

The best sportswear brands now produce clothing with many 'technical' qualities to make your workout more comfortable. Fabrics are designed to be:

★ **Lightweight** – so there's less to carry;

★ **Breathable** – to allow body heat to escape;

★ **Wicking** – to lift sweat away from the body and prevent clothes from becoming soaked;

★ **Waterproof** – to keep the rain out;

★ **Windproof** – to prevent cold winds chilling you.

If you can afford it, technical fabrics can make your workouts more comfortable, but never feel you can't train because you haven't got the latest clothing. Basic cotton T-shirts and sweatshirts are also great and if you worry too much about how you look then you're probably not focused enough on your workout. If you can afford just one item, then go for a lightweight waterproof running jacket for your outdoor workouts. These are designed to be waterproof and windproof and yet ultra-lightweight and they will keep you warm and dry in most conditions.

WATER BOTTLE

It is essential that you drink water throughout your workouts. You can simply carry a small mineral water bottle. There are also several sports bottles available, designed to be easy to carry during a workout – either fitting round your waist or slotting over your fingers so you can run and walk with your hand relaxed rather than clenched.

4 WHERE WILL YOU WORK OUT?

OUTDOORS

The ever-changing terrain and wind resistance mean that exercising outdoors will always be more of a challenge than indoor-based workouts. Plus, outdoors there is no big red button to push that says 'stop' if you feel like giving up halfway through your run – you still have to get home. Give up halfway through a treadmill run and it's an easy stroll to the changing rooms.

Ideally, you should do your morning Pyramid Powerwalk/Jog outdoors, preferably in a green space where you are away from traffic pollution. With the right kit (see pages 51–53) you should be able to do this whatever the weather. If you really don't have anywhere suitable to work out outdoors, then you can do your Pyramid Powerwalk/Jog on a treadmill indoors. In this case, set it at a 5% incline to simulate the wind and terrain resistance you get outdoors.

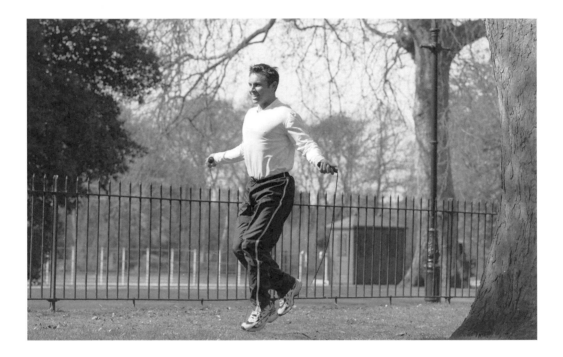

GYM V HOME

Your Upper and Lower Body Power Circuits are designed to be done at home or in a gym. The circuits in Week 1 are perfect for doing at home since the only equipment you need is a barbell set. In Week 2, you have the option of either continuing to work out at home or taking your workout into a gym. You may want to do this if you feel motivated by working in a group environment, if you're already paying for a gym membership or if you don't have the space or privacy at home. Each circuit includes options for weight training machines if you prefer to work out this way rather than using the barbell. It also allows you to add some variety into the program so you don't have to do the same thing day in, day out.

Your Home Gym Equipment

The exercise equipment industry is huge and there are more and more state-of-the-art machines on sale every year. A lot are highly computerised and very expensive. But do you need such equipment? The fittest people you can hope to meet are in the military and the style of training they rely on uses the same basic, traditional equipment that has been used for years. With just the following 3 pieces of equipment, you can get fit and stay fit for the rest of your life.

★ **Barbell with basic weights set.** This can be bought at a good department store or sports store for around £40 ($56). The barbell will come with a basic set of plates that will be suitable for the exercises in the program.
★ **Dumbbell set.** As above, a basic dumbbell set with a range of weights can be bought from sports stores or department stores. A system like the PowerBlock dumbbell system gives you a whole set of dumbbell weights in a stackable, space-saving format.
★ **Adjustable exercise bench.** This is used to perform many exercises from standing and seated positions – it is adjustable from flat to vertical.

5 WORK OUT YOUR STARTING STATE OF FITNESS

In the military, everyone must pass the Basic Fitness Test (BFT) before they are accepted. This BFT is your personal 'quality assessment' (QA) – a regular part of military life. It is used to measure, compare and keep track of your physical fitness and how you are improving.

Do the BFT before you start the program, 2 weeks into the program and at the very end of the program. Fill in your results on the chart on page 57 and you will have an instant visual record of your progress. You can repeat this process at regular intervals after you have completed the 30-day program to check on your progress.

MEASUREMENTS

Measuring your body is a far more accurate record of body shape improvements than weighing yourself. You will lose body fat on this program but it may not register on the scales because you'll also be building lean muscle tissue, which weighs more than fat (but it takes up less space, so you'll look leaner).

Use a tape measure to record the circumference of your chest, upper arm, waist, hips and upper thigh. Then simply re-measure and record every 2 weeks.

SIT-UPS

Record how many basic crunches you can do with good slow technique until you can do no more (*see* page 74 for how to do the perfect crunch). This will measure your abdominal strength and stamina. No stopping and restarting is allowed.

PRESS-UPS

Record how many full or half press-ups you can do with good technique (*see* pages 83–4 for how to do the perfect press-up). This measures upper body strength. Start with full press-ups if you can, continuing on your knees until you can go no further.

STANDING JUMP TEST

Stand next to a wall with chalk on your fingers. Bend your knees and jump as high as you can, touching the wall at your highest point. Record the measurement. This measures your athletic ability.

RECOVERY HEART RATE

Powerwalk 1½ miles or for 15 minutes. Run back or alternate run/walking. Rest for 30 seconds then take your pulse for 6 seconds. Times the result by 10. This is your recovery heart rate. The lower it is – the faster your heart recovers from exertion – the stronger and fitter it is. (You know your heart is in good shape when the figure is about 75–84 or less).

Your Personal Fitness Record

	★ Test 1 ★ Date:	★ Test 2 ★ Date:	★ Test 3 ★ Date:
Chest measurement			
Arm measurement			
Waist measurement			
Hip measurement			
Thigh measurement			
Number of sit-ups			
Number of press-ups			
Standing jump test			
Recovery heart rate			

CHAPTER 5: KEY POINTS

★ Think carefully about when you start your 30 days – choose a period of time in which you're most likely to be able to follow the program without missing any days.

★ Make sure you're in optimum health before you start the program.

★ Get the right equipment in place.

★ Do your Basic Fitness Test and record your results.

★ Keep focused and motivated – your enthusiasm should be high.

TRAINING ZONES:

HOW TO EXERCISE
AT THE RIGHT LEVEL

How do you know if you are doing too much or too little work when you train? If you are experienced you will be familiar with the way you feel when you work at different levels of intensity – but if you are new to training then you'll need to discover your zones by paying attention to how your body responds to different activities.

Even if you already work out on a regular basis, don't think about skipping this section. All too often, people who are following a long-term fitness plan will 'plateau' once they reach a comfortable level of fitness. If your workouts stop being a challenge they can become less rewarding and eventually no fun at all. Remember that real success and personal reward come from continually pushing your personal barriers. Intensity zones are a good way to ensure you work hard enough while staying within the safe training zones.

The Commando Workout is designed for everyone from an absolute beginner to a committed 5-times-a-week exerciser. The interval training system will ensure that you will have the opportunity to push yourself to new limits, whatever your starting point.

SETTING YOUR PERSONAL INTENSITY ZONE

Each exercise session will involve working at different levels, from 1–10. These levels are personal to you and allow you to customize the workouts for maximum effectiveness.

Setting your personal intensity zone is about working with the 'Rate of Perceived Exertion' (RPE). This is a way of tracking your heartbeat and lung output by using physical signs rather than a heart-rate monitor or other equipment. It is about recognising your personal levels so that when the program asks you to work at a particular level, you know when you have reached it.

Here's how each level should feel to you:

Level 1: Total Rest	Total rest, as when you are asleep or relaxing on couch.
Level 2: Minimal Moving	Minimal activity – sitting at a desk working.
Level 3: Relaxed Effort	The equivalent of gentle walking – you should feel slightly warmer.
Level 4: Switched on	The equivalent of purposeful walking. Your heart rate is starting to rise and you're feeling warmer. You begin to 'glow' rather than sweat.
Level 5: Starting to Work	Your activity should now feel moderate. You feel warm and you're starting to sweat but you can still carry out a full conversation.
Level 6: A Steady Workout	Your breathing gets heavier and carrying on a conversation requires effort – although it is still possible to talk.
Levels 7–8: Working Hard	Working conversation is reduced to words rather than sentences. You are sweating and hot. Your activity should feel 'hard'.
Levels 9–10: Maximum Effort	You can no longer talk. After a short period at this level you will feel like your lungs are bursting and your heart is beating at its maximum. It's not a comfortable place to be for any length of time – your brain will be sending you frantic messages to slow down. And you will.

THE PYRAMID TRAINING TECHNIQUE

Your Pyramid Powerwalks/Jogs and Power Circuits are designed around a pyramid structure. This means that you start off at a comfortable pace, then gradually pick it up until you reach a peak around halfway through the workout. Then you gradually bring it back down to resting again.

This pyramid structure, reaching a peak in the middle of your workout, is the key to the success of the program. By working the heart, lungs and muscles at such an intense level, even for a short period, the body is forced to make adaptations that make it more efficient. It also increases the number of calories you burn per session and produces an 'afterburn' effect in which your metabolic rate is raised – burning more calories – for up to 18 hours after your exercise session. This is one of the reasons why your nutrition is so important.

When you exercise at Levels 9–10, you are entering the 'anaerobic threshold'. Up to this point the exercise has been aerobic, meaning 'in the presence of oxygen'. The energy to fuel your Powerwalk/Jog has come from the oxidation (burning with oxygen) of fat and carbohydrate. But once you reach Levels 9–10, the body can't use oxygen fast enough to convert these products to energy, so it shifts to anaerobic, or non-oxidative, energy pro- duction. A bi-product of this process is the accumulation of lactic acid in the muscles, a sign that you are using energy up faster than it can be produced. (Contrary to popular belief, this isn't entirely a waste product – the body can convert lactic acid back to energy when you are recovering from your workout).

Reaching your anaerobic threshold doesn't feel great – your breathing becomes laboured and uncomfortable, your muscles start to burn and your brain will be scream- ing at you to stop. This is why the program only expects you to be working at this level for a short period of time, but it is the part of your training program that will help you gain the most results and will help you train comfortably at a harder intensity. That means burning the maximum number of calories in the minimum amount of time – exactly what you want.

The Pyramid Training Technique

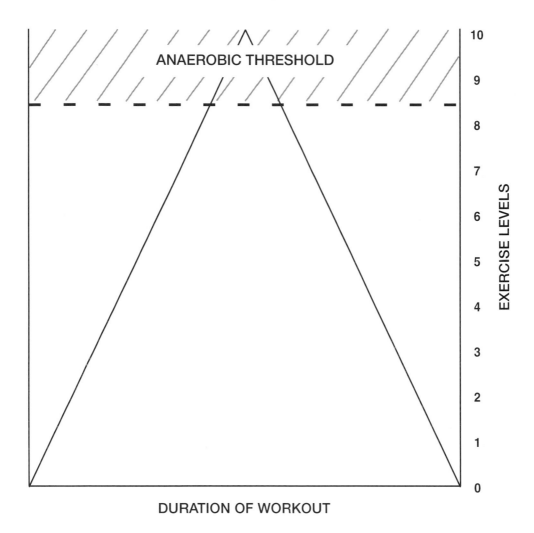

It also means that your cardiovascular training will start to feel easier with time – you'll feel tired less quickly and recover faster. Ever done the same run 3 times a week and wondered why after 6 weeks or so it still doesn't feel any easier? That's because if you don't challenge your body each time, pushing it to work as hard as you can – even for as short a time as a couple of minutes – it will never grow stronger. Don't forget that a stronger heart is also more efficient at delivering oxygen to every cell in your body, so it will even make your weight training sessions feel easier.

Healthwise, here's what you can gain from conditioning your cardiovascular system in this way:

★ Reduced risk of heart disease and stroke;
★ Decreased cholesterol levels;
★ Reduced blood pressure;
★ Decreased body fat;
★ Decreased risk of diabetes;
★ More efficient delivery of blood and oxygen, so increasing general energy levels;
★ Better efficiency at getting rid of waste products.

WHY PEAK IN THE MIDDLE?

In some training plans, you work at a steady pace until the very last few minutes of the session when you push yourself as hard as you can. But do you have enough energy left at the end of a session really to do this justice? The commando-style pyramid workout means:

★ You do your hardest work when your muscles are fully warmed up.
★ You push yourself when you still have the energy to really give it your best shot.
★ Your workout is maximally efficient so will give you better results – you are testing yourself.
★ The last part of the workout, where you gradually bring your intensity levels back down, feels like a breeze in comparison!
★ You are more likely to have the confidence to complete the full session every time.

POWER CIRCUITS

The weight training sessions included in your 4-week program are designed as circuits – a series of exercises performed consecutively in quick succession. This is the optimal way to improve overall muscle tone and strength as well as muscle stamina and endurance.

Muscle strength is the amount of force a muscle can produce – in other words, the amount of weight it can lift. Muscle endurance is the ability of a muscle to continue contracting against a resistance – to carry out a repetitive workload for a period of time.

The amount of strength and endurance your muscles develop – and whether they develop more of one than the other – depends on the type of workouts you do. Different activities will promote the development of the 'slow twitch' and 'fast twitch' muscle fibres. Your Power Circuits are designed to develop your capabilities for both types of muscle with 'explosive' and 'endurance' activities.

Slow twitch fibres are your building blocks for endurance. As the name suggests, they contract relatively slowly. They have many capillaries (ensuring a steady supply of oxygenating blood) and mitochondria (the power houses of cells) and are used in aerobic activities such as jogging, middle- and long-distance running and walking. Fast twitch muscle fibres are used in 'explosive' strength work. They have relatively poor endurance and are used for explosive power activities like sprinting and jumping.

As with your morning PowerWalk/Jog, your Power Circuits are designed so you peak in the middle, when your muscles are fully warmed up but still have the energy to perform the exercises with the best technique and truly reach your peak.

CHAPTER 6: KEY POINTS

★ The key to the program is pushing yourself as hard as you can for a short period of time in the middle of your workout.

★ Quality, not quantity gets results – a short workout which challenges your body is better than a long one that doesn't.

★ The rate you work out throughout each session is personal to you and depends on your individual fitness levels.

★ Learning to recognise your personal exertion levels is the key to exercising at the right rate to get results.

★ Constantly push yourself, pushing your limits.

★ Always train smart. A smart trainer is a results-orientated trainer.

PREPARATION AND RECOVERY

If you value your fitness and don't want to pick up injuries, you will take the time to allow your body to prepare and recover from exercise. A gradual warm-up and, later on, a cool-down – including stretching out those muscles you have just worked – may not be a 'hard' part of your session, but is vital to the development of your strength and endurance.

The warm-up phase is designed gradually to increase the flow of blood and oxygen to the muscles, and to raise the heart rate and basic body temperature. This enables your muscles to contract more easily so you can work at a higher rate and with far less chance of 'pulling' or tearing something. Warming up also encourages the flow of synovial fluid to the joints, so your range of movement and joint flexibility will be increased before you start. Warming up also makes the rest of your workout feel easier and helps you to perform better.

You wouldn't expect your car to go from freezing cold to 60 mph in a matter of seconds without damaging it, so don't make unrealistic demands on your body. Without a warm-up and cool-down, even if you don't think you are hurting yourself, you are reducing the overall effectiveness of your workout and greatly increasing the risk of long term injury.

It's for these reasons that professional athletes think nothing of warming up for up to 45–60 minutes before a training session. I'm not suggesting you go that far, but a 5-minute warm-up will make a big difference both to your cardiovascular and your weight training sessions.

WARMING UP

This doesn't have to be complicated or time consuming. At its simplest level, a warm-up is a 5-minute walk or slow jog, perhaps incorporating some shoulder or arm rolls to loosen up your upper body. If you're about to do your weight training session in the gym, then spend 5 minutes on a rowing machine, treadmill or exercise bike. If you're doing your workout at home, then you could try skipping at a moderate pace for 5 minutes, or simply marching on the spot.

Some workout programs include stretches at this point, but recent research suggests that stretching before your muscles are fully warm (when you have really worked them) is of little real benefit. It is after your workout that stretching becomes most important.

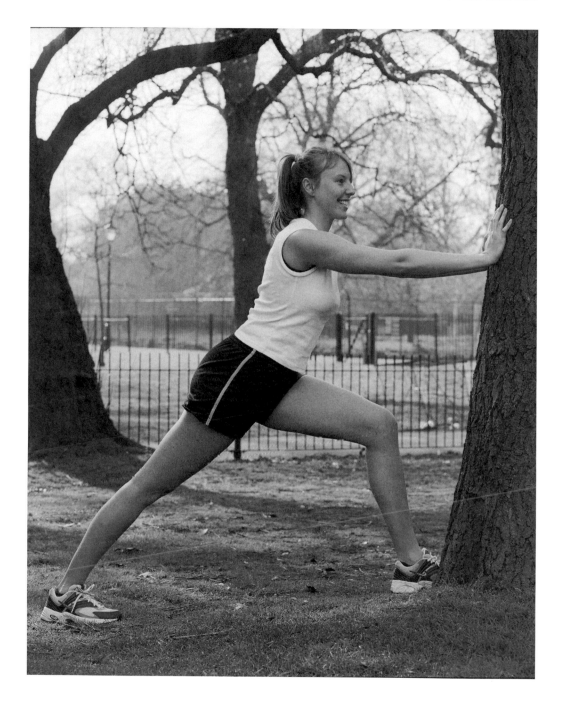

COOLING DOWN AND STRETCHING OUT

Ending your workout abruptly can lead to pooling of the blood and sluggish circulation, and it will increase the chances of feeling sore and stiff the next day. Cooling down, by walking or jogging at a moderate pace for 5 minutes, will also safely return your heart rate to a normal level.

The end of your workout is the ideal time to improve your flexibility by stretching. Don't think flexibility is only useful for ballet dancers – it can improve both your strength and endurance training. For example, most runners notice that their calf and hamstring muscles (at the back of the thighs) become tight after a while which can shorten the stride and reduce speed. Reduced flexibility can also limit the range of movement during strength exercises and this means that the muscle isn't fully challenged, so your strength development will slow right down.

HOW TO STRETCH

The following stretch sequences target every muscle group in your body. You should learn these sequences so that they become second nature. Hold each stretch for 30 seconds then flow straight to the next stretch in the sequence.

When you stretch, sometimes you may feel what I describe as a 'comfortable pain', at other times you may feel very little. Stretching prevents injury to the muscle and reduces muscle soreness.

THE UPPER BODY SEQUENCE

All the following stretches are done standing with feet shoulder-width apart.

NECK

Gently tilt the head to one side until you feel a stretch on the opposite side of the neck. Repeat tilting your head to the other side.

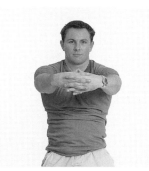

UPPER BACK

Clasp your hands together and push your arms straight out in front of you at shoulder level.

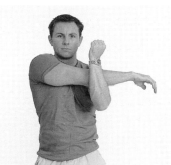

CHEST

Hold your abdominals tight and keep your head, neck and shoulders relaxed. Clasp your hands behind your back and lift your arms behind you until you feel the stretch across your chest.

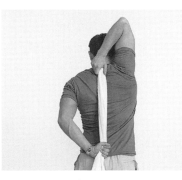

SHOULDERS

Bend one arm and bring it across your body at shoulder height. Place your opposite hand or forearm on the upper arm and push to increase the stretch. Repeat on the other side.

TRICEPS

Raise one arm in the air, bend at the elbow and place the hand in the middle of your shoulder blades. Use the opposite hand to push against your arm to increase the stretch. Repeat on the other side. Alternatively, use a towel to increase the stretch, as left.

THE LOWER BODY SEQUENCE

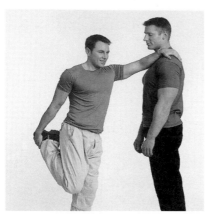

QUADS (FRONT THIGHS) AND HIPS

Stand up straight with one hand on a wall, chair or a friend to support you. Bend one leg back behind you, pulling your foot to your buttock and keeping your knees together. Repeat on the other leg.

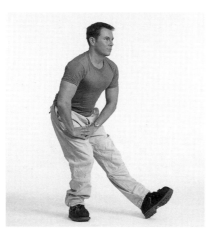

HAMSTRING (BACK THIGHS)

Stand with one leg in front of the other so it is straight out in front of you. Bend your supporting leg slightly then bend forward from the hips. Repeat on the other leg.

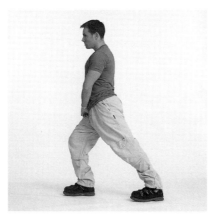

CALVES

Stand in front of a wall or bench using both hands to support you. Step back with one foot behind you. Keep your front leg slightly bent and the back leg straight. Push the heel of your back leg into the ground. Repeat on the other leg.

GLUTES (BUTTOCKS)

Lie on your back with both legs bent and feet flat on the floor. Then lift one foot and rest it just above the knee on the thigh of the other leg. Grasp the same thigh with both hands and pull the leg towards you. Repeat on the other side.

ACHIEVING CORE STRENGTH – WORKING YOUR ABDOMINAL MUSCLES

Most men and women rate a '6 pack' or at least having flat abs as one of their goals when they work out. However, from a strength and fitness perspective there are more important reasons than 'definition' and 'flatness' as to why you should put effort into training your abdominal region.

The muscles that make up your torso are your foundation of fitness – if they are strong, every other movement will feel easier. Strong abdominals also ward off the risk of back pain in the future. Many of the resistance exercises in this 4-week program will work the abdominals, as will your Powerwalk/Jog, but there are also some specific exercises to add to target this area. It's up to you when you fit them in, but you should aim to do them at least 3 times a week. Here's a few suggestions how:

★ Do them in the morning after your Powerwalk/Jog and before your full body stretches
★ Do them before your PM Power Circuit but after the warm-up
★ Do them after your PM Power Circuit but before your cool-down stretches.

YOUR ESSENTIAL AB EXERCISES

Aim to complete 3 sets of 25 reps of each exercise or do as many as you can with good technique. Stop as soon as you feel your technique is suffering – when muscles other than your abs, such as your neck or thighs (hip flexors), are doing the work. Always exhale on the up or exertion part of the exercises for full contraction of the abs.

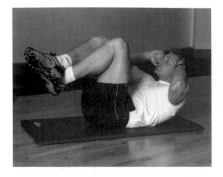

CRUNCHES – LEGS UP

Lie on your back with your legs in the air and your hands by your ears. Bend your knees and curl your legs towards your ribcage as you curl your shoulders forwards. Don't pull on your neck. Hold for 2 seconds then return to the start position.

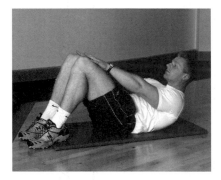

CRUNCHES – FEET FLAT

Lie on your back with your knees bent, feet flat on the floor and hands by your knees. Curl your shoulders forwards, keeping your lower back on the floor and your abdominals pulled in. Keep a space the size of a fist between your chin and chest to ensure your head stays in line with your spine. Hold then return to the start position.

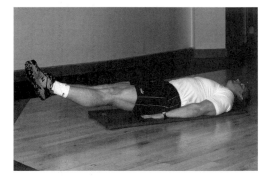

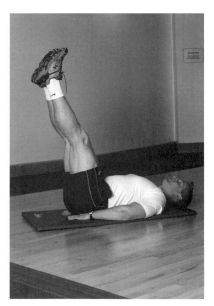

LEG RAISES

Lie on your back with your hands by your sides and your legs in the air. Tighten your lower abdominals and lift your hips, raising your legs straight up. Hold and return to the start position.

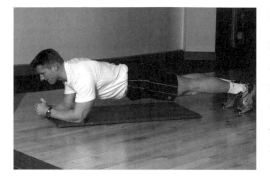

PLANK (ADVANCED EXERCISERS ONLY)

Start with your body face to the ground, supported on your toes and elbows. There should be a straight line from your shoulders to your ankles. Pull in your abdominals but don't let your bottom stick in the air. Hold for as long as you can.

ALTERNATE ELBOWS TO KNEE

This works your obliques even more than your abs. Lie back with your legs in the air. Cross your elbow over to the opposite knee. Repeat to the other side.

When doing your ab exercises, remember the following important points:

1   All the exercises should be completed with perfect form and execution.
2   Try to complete 25 reps of each exercise and repeat the cycle 3 times.
3   To create more intensity, hold the top part of each rep for a few seconds before releasing.
4   Don't rush to get through them.

Fiction: The reason it is called a 6-pack is because it is 6 different muscles.
Fact: It is all one muscle but it looks like 6 because it is split by the ligaments.
You work all the muscle all the time – there is no upper, middle and lower ab muscle. You may put a little more stress on the upper or lower fibres but every rep is working all the muscle.

Fiction: Doing a lot of stomach work will reduce your stomach and flatten it.
Fact: Yes, you are training the muscle and toning it, but not reducing your stomach.
Some people work their stomachs all their lives, but they burn no fat so they never get to see a 6-pack.

CHAPTER 7: KEYPOINTS

★   Never skip your warm-up – it helps you perform better.
★   Train your abs 3 times at week.

Chapter Eight

YOUR 4-WEEK PROGRAM

TO COMMANDO FITNESS

You should now be ready to start your 4-week program. You should feel excited and ready to take on the challenge. If you feel a bit daunted then that's good too – it means you have accepted that you are going to do something that's a bit different, a bit new and challenging!

WEEK 1 TRAINING PROGRAM

	Day 1	Day 2	Day 3
AM	Powerwalk/Jog	Powerwalk/Jog	Powerwalk/Jog
PM	Upper Body Power Circuit	Lower Body Power Circuit	Rest and Recovery

Although you will be planning ahead, preparing your kit, your agenda and your diary for your challenge, one thing you should not do is get too caught up in the idea that you've got '4 weeks of work' ahead. Be prepared, but don't start out thinking you've got a mountain in your way – just remember that all journeys start with a single step. Keep your focus in the present and before you know it you'll be well under way, feeling fitter and stronger than ever before.

Day 4	Day 5	Day 6	Day 7
Rest and Recovery	Powerwalk/Jog	Powerwalk/Jog	ACTIVE REST DAY
Upper Body Power Circuit	Lower Body Power Circuit	Upper Body Power Circuit	

Remember, the world is full of heroes and you can be one too. Make today the start of the rest of your life – if you don't ever try, you will never know how great you can be. In my time in the military I have seen many feats of bravery accomplished by ordinary men and women and I know that when given the opportunity everyone, even the least expected, can rise to new strengths. This is your opportunity – so take it, relish it and see yourself rise to the challenge.

WEEK 1 – DAY 1

Start with a positive mental attitude. Your PM Power Circuit will build muscle strength and endurance in your shoulders (deltoids), arms (biceps, triceps), back (lats), chest (pectorals), and will use core abdominal strength too. Let's do it!

AM – PYRAMID POWERWALK/JOG

Equipment needed: watch/stopwatch, water bottle.

PM – UPPER BODY POWER CIRCUIT

Equipment needed: barbell, chair or bench for the shoulder press and triceps dip and, ideally, a mirror to watch your technique throughout.

AM – PYRAMID POWERWALK/JOG

As explained in Chapter 6 (*see* pages 62-4), your Pyramid Powerwalk/Jog is designed so that you start off at a comfortable pace, then gradually ease into working harder until you reach a peak right in the middle of your workout. You then gradually bring the pace back down again.

Your Rates of Perceived Exertion (RPE) are personal to you. Depending on your fitness levels, your level 9 or 10, the ultimate challenge for your muscles and your heart and lungs, may be a very fast walk. But if you are already fit, you may need to break into a run to reach your peak. If you already run regularly, you'll have started jogging from the beginning of the workout to reach Level 5 and will need to sprint to reach your Level 9.

Don't think you're taking the 'soft option' if you choose to powerwalk instead of jog. For years, powerwalking – or 'yomping' – has formed the foundation of military fitness.

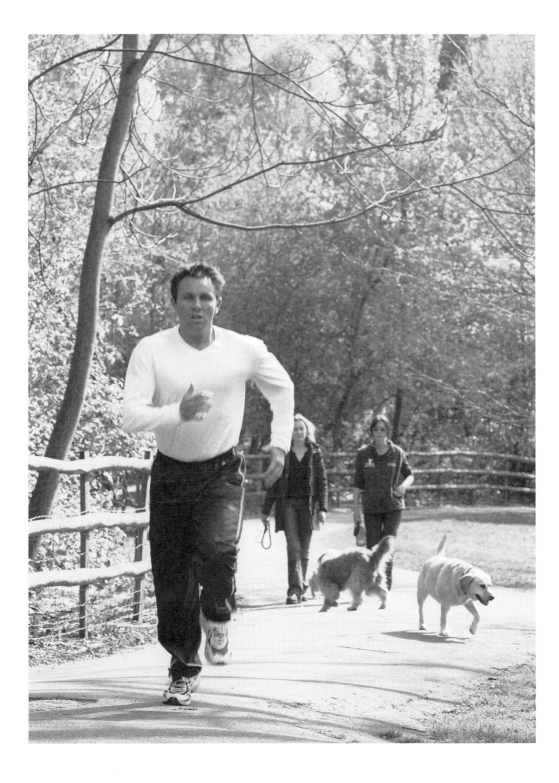

On a practical level, this mix of very fast walking and short bursts of running is the fastest way to cover long distances, particularly when carrying a heavy backpack. It is used because it is possible to sustain it for hours at a time and also because it places much less impact on the joints than running. Plus, yomping or fast walking involves the upper body much more than running does, so you're getting a more balanced work out.

Doing the Pyramid Powerwalk/Jog

OK, so here we go. You've got the motivation and determination, what next?

5 minutes warm-up at level 3
2½ minutes at level 5
2½ minutes at level 6
2½ minutes at level 7
2½ minutes at level 8
2½ minutes at level 9
2½ minutes at level 8
2½ minutes at level 7
2½ minutes at level 6
5 minutes cool-down at level 3.

Complete the full body stretches (*see* pages 70–72). Don't forget to drink water throughout, sipping rather than gulping. (*See* page 61 for how to measure your effort levels.)

PM – UPPER BODY POWER CIRCUIT

Equipment needed: Barbell, chair or bench for the shoulder press and triceps dip and, ideally, a mirror to watch your technique throughout.

How to choose the weight: Fit the weight on your barbell that allows you to do 12 biceps curls, but no more – the last 2 repetitions (reps) should be challenging.

Press-ups

Start with your weight on your hands and feet, and your hands directly under your shoulders, keeping your back and legs straight. Bend your arms and lower your body until your chest is a couple of inches off the ground (if you're working with a partner, they should be able to fit their fist between your chest and the floor). Keep your back straight and don't stick your bottom in the air. Breathe in, then press back up to the start position while breathing out.

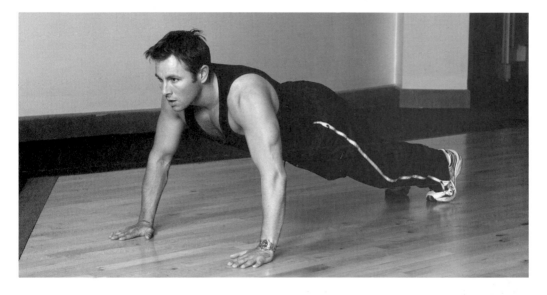

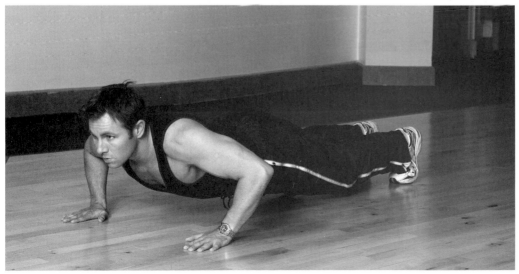

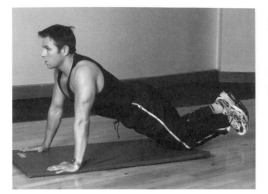

Alternative: Half press-up

Your arms are in the same position as above, but your weight rests on the soft part of your knees, not your feet.

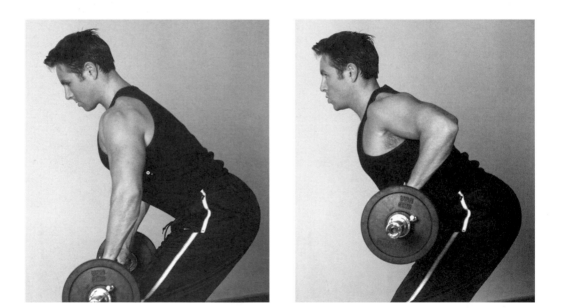

Bentover row

Stand with your feet shoulder-width apart, knees bent. Bend from the waist, keeping your back flat, and hold the barbell with straight arms in front of your shins. Breathing out, pull the barbell up to your stomach by squeezing your shoulder blades, pulling your arms close to your sides. Hold for 2 seconds then return to the start position.

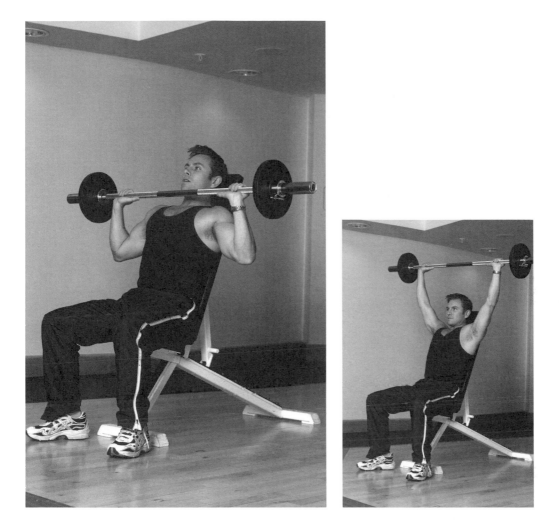

Shoulder press

Sitting on a chair or bench with your back well supported and your feet hip-width apart, hold the barbell above your head so your arms are bent at a 90-degree angle and your elbows are level with your shoulders. Press the bar upwards by raising your arms above your head. Hold for 1 second then return to the start position. Never lock out your elbows – keep the tension on the muscle.

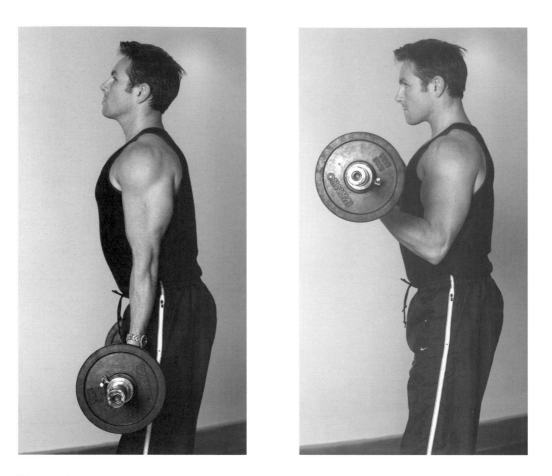

Bicep curls

Stand with your feet hip-width apart and knees soft. Start with your arms by your sides, elbows slightly bent, holding the barbell in front of you so your palms face away from your body. Slowly raise the barbell to your chest, keeping your elbows tucked in close to your body. Squeeze your biceps then return to the start position.

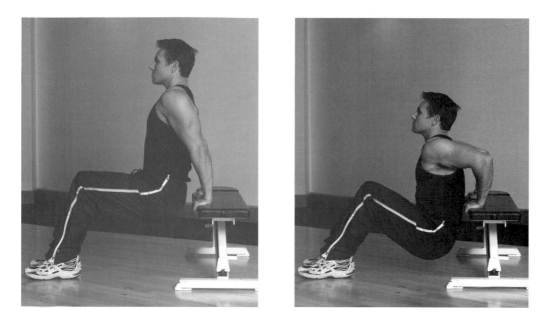

Tricep dips

Standing with your back to the chair or bench, bend your legs and place your hands on the front edge of the bench, facing forward. Position your feet in front of you so most of the weight is on your arms. Keeping your elbows tucked against the sides of the body, lower your body until your upper arms are parallel with the floor. Your hips should drop straight down to a couple of inches off the floor and your back should stay close to the bench. Return to the start position by straightening your arms. Don't lock out your elbows.

DOING THE UPPER BODY POWER CIRCUIT

Do the exercises in the order specified, moving quickly from one exercise to the next, following this sequence:

  5 reps of each exercise, 1 minute rest
  8 reps of each exercise, 1 minute rest
  15 reps of each exercise, 1 minute rest
  8 reps of each exercise, 1 minute rest
  5 reps of each exercise, 1 minute rest.

Each individual move should be slow and controlled – do them at speed and gravity will do too much of the work. Follow your session with the upper body stretches (*see* pages 70–71).

GOAL	COMPLETED
30-min powerwalk/jog	
Press-ups 5–8–15–8–5	
Bentover row 5–8–15–8–5	
Shoulder press 5–8–15–8–5	
Bicep curls 5–8–15–8–5	
Tricep dips 5–8–15–8–5	
Effort level	
Energy	
Enjoyment	
Overall performance	
COMMENTS:	

FOOD LOG	
FOOD EATEN	TIME EATEN

Estimated water consumption

COMMENTS:

WEEK 1 – DAY 2

Today's Power Circuit focuses on the muscles that work your legs. These include your quads (front of legs), hamstrings (back of legs), glutes (bottom) and calves (lower leg). These are the strongest muscles in your body and you will find that the weights you use are slightly heavier than for your upper body circuit.

AM – PYRAMID POWERWALK/JOG

PM – LOWER BODY POWER CIRCUIT

Equipment needed: Bench for step-ups, barbell for dead lifts.

PM – LOWER BODY POWER CIRCUIT

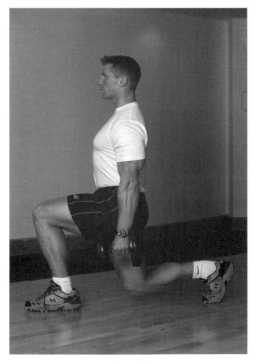

Lunges

Start with both legs together, then stride forward a good pace with your right. Bend both knees to lower your body until your right thigh is parallel with the floor. Push on the thigh muscles of both legs to return to the start position and repeat stepping out with your left leg. When stepping back, push through your heel not your toes. For an extra challenge, hold a dumbbell in each hand.

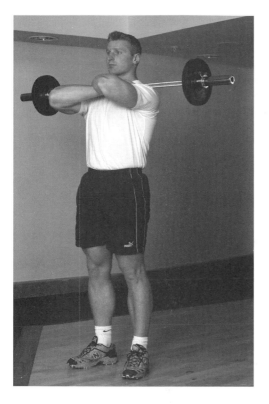

Front squats

Stand with your feet hip-width apart, knees slightly bent. Keeping your back straight but allowing your body to lean forwards slightly, sit back as if you were sitting in a chair, bending your knees until your thighs are parallel with the floor. Don't let your knees move over the line of your toes. Hold and push back to the start position without locking out your knees. For an extra challenge, hold your barbell across your shoulders.

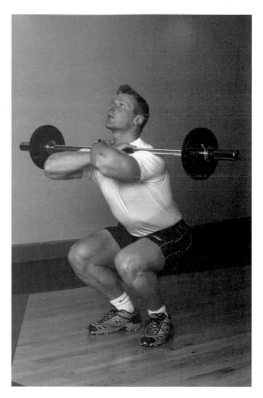

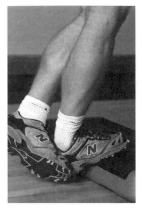 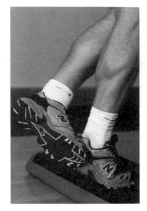

Calf raises

Stand facing a wall, about half an arm's length away with your hands resting flat on the wall for balance. Raise your left foot off the floor. Now rise up on to the toe of your right foot, keeping the leg straight. Return to the start position then repeat with your left leg. To add resistance, fill a backpack with some bottles of water and wear it on your back.

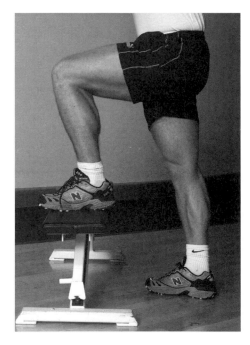 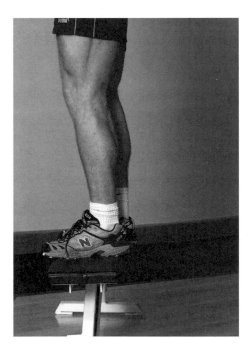

Step-ups

Stand facing the bench. Step up with one foot, keeping your back straight and placing your whole foot on the bench. Step up with the other foot then step down, one foot at a time. Make sure that you use alternate legs to step up with each time.

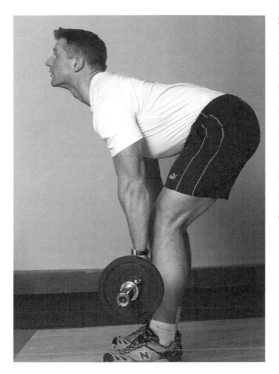

Straight-leg dead lift

Stand up straight with your feet shoulder-width apart, holding the barbell with your palms facing your thighs. Bend forwards at the hips then slowly lower the barbell until it nearly reaches the floor. Keep your upper back straight – don't hunch over. Return to the start position, bringing your hips through at the end.

DOING THE LOWER BODY POWER CIRCUIT

Do the exercises in the order specified, moving quickly from one exercise to the next, following this sequence. Be sure to be fluent and keep the continuity going.

10 reps of each exercise, 1 minute rest
15 reps of each exercise, 1 minute rest
20 reps of each exercise, 1 minute rest
15 reps of each exercise, 1 minute rest
10 reps of each exercise, 1 minute rest.

Each individual move should be deliberate and controlled at a medium pace. (A medium pace is for a count of 2 up and 2 down.) Where an exercise uses the left and right legs separately, you have completed one rep when you've done both sides. Finish with the lower body stretches (*see* page 72–3).

GOAL	COMPLETED
30-min powerwalk/jog	
Front squats 10–15–20–15–10	
Lunges 10–15–20–15–10	
Calf raises 10–15–20–15–10	
Step-ups 10–15–20–15–10	
Straight-leg dead lifts 10–15–20–15–10	
Effort level	
Energy	
Enjoyment	
Overall performance	
COMMENTS:	

FOOD LOG	
FOOD EATEN	**TIME EATEN**
Estimated water consumption	
COMMENTS:	

WEEK 1 – DAY 3

Today, your evening session is Rest and Recovery time to allow your muscles the time out they require to respond and adapt to the work you did in the Power Circuits. Ensure you use the time to fuel up with food and a lot of water.

AM – PYRAMID POWERWALK/JOG

PM – REST AND RECOVERY

AM – PYRAMID POWERWALK/JOG

Be proud of yourself. You are well on the way now and there is no turning back!

☆ TECHNIQUE TIP ☆ POWERWALKING

What's the difference between a walk and a powerwalk? In powerwalking, you move so fast that it would be easier to start jogging – in fact, your body has to work to stop you from breaking into a run. You walk at the speed you would if you were 10 minutes late for a very important appointment – you should cover around 2–3 miles in your 30-minute session. Try to keep the following in mind when you walk:

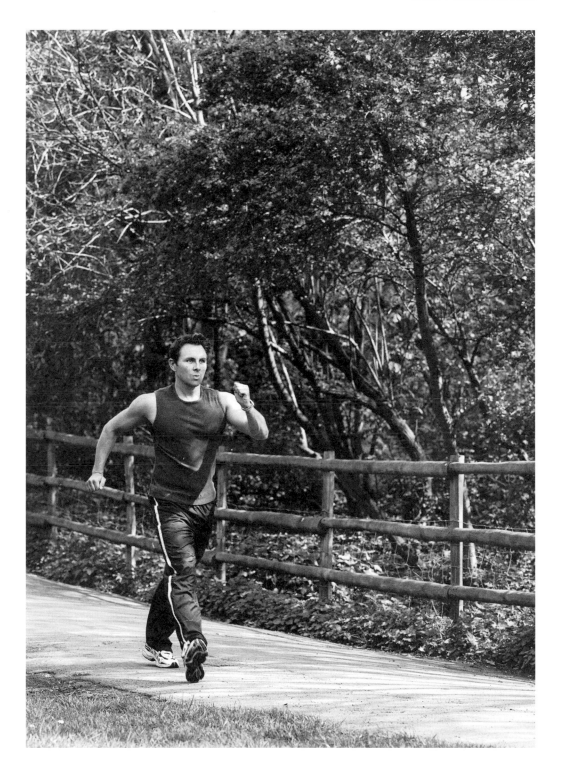

★ **Head** – keep your head up and neck relaxed. Look ahead of you, not down at the ground, as this would put pressure on your neck and spine

★ **Arms** – bend your elbows at 90 degrees. Hands should be loose, never clenched. Don't 'chicken wing' – keep your elbows close to your body. Keep your arms moving at waist height – pumping your arms high in the air is a waste of energy

★ **Hips** – your hips should rotate front to back with each stride, not side to side. You don't have to develop an exaggerated hip motion; it should come naturally as part of a good stride

★ **Legs** – don't overstride by taking longer steps in front of your body. Keep your stride length natural, but learn to use it powerfully. Your stride should be longer behind your body than in front – the force of the stride comes from pushing off your back foot and engaging the power of your hamstrings (back of thigh muscles) and gluteals (buttock muscles). Add speed by increasing the number of strides you take rather than trying to lengthen your stride

★ **Feet** – strike the ground first with your heel, ankle flexed. Someone standing in front of you should be able to see the sole of your foot with every step. Roll through the step from heel to toe. Always push off forcefully from the toe of the foot behind your body.

GOAL	COMPLETED
30-min powerwalk/jog	
Effort level	
Energy	
Enjoyment	
Overall performance	
COMMENTS:	

FOOD LOG	
FOOD EATEN	**TIME EATEN**
Estimated water consumption	

COMMENTS:

WEEK 1 – DAY 4

Today, your morning session is a rest period. Running, jogging and powerwalking all put stress on your joints and resting them now will benefit you in the long term. Enjoy yourself and eat well!

AM – REST AND RECOVERY

PM – UPPER BODY POWER CIRCUIT

AM – UPPER BODY POWER CIRCUIT

☆ TECHNIQUE TIP ☆   GETTING THE TECHNIQUE RIGHT

How can two people spend the same time exercising and doing the same activities every week, and one lose more weight and look leaner than the other? It is not just a case of life being unfair, differing metabolic rates or genetics. Technique – how you carry out your activities – is often the key that makes the difference between getting the results you want and never quite making it. Do an exercise incorrectly, and however many reps you complete, it won't get you the desired results. Exercising with poor technique can also put your body at risk of injury.

Detailed instructions are included in this book for every exercise. You'll reap a multitude of benefits by investing enough time to practise and get the technique right. Exercising in front of a mirror or getting a friend to watch you can help.

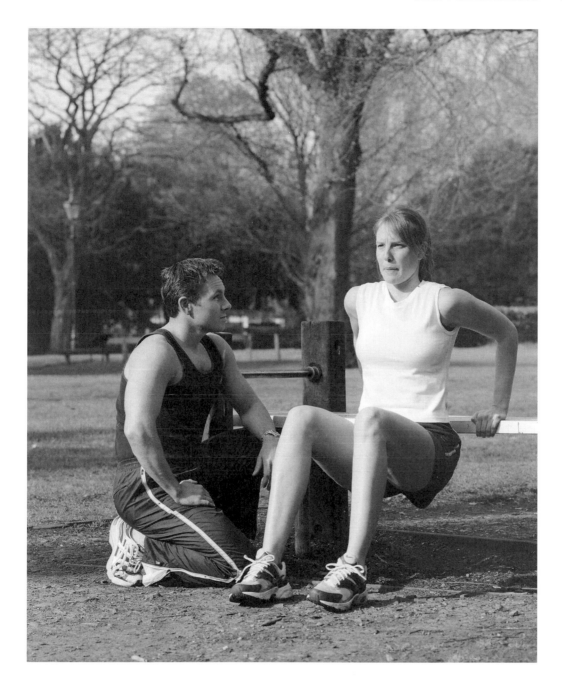

GOAL		COMPLETED
Press-ups 5–8–15–8–5		
Bentover row 5–8–15–8–5		
Shoulder press 5–8–15–8–5		
Bicep curls 5–8–15–8–5		
Tricep dips 5–8–15–8–5		
Effort level		
Energy		
Enjoyment		
Overall performance		
COMMENTS:		

FOOD LOG	
FOOD EATEN	**TIME EATEN**
Estimated water consumption	
COMMENTS:	

WEEK 1 – DAY 5

Today's sessions are both familiar to you now. Can you do them better than you did the first time?

> **AM – PYRAMID POWERWALK/JOG**
>
> **PM – LOWER BODY POWER CIRCUIT**

AM – PYRAMID POWERWALK/JOG

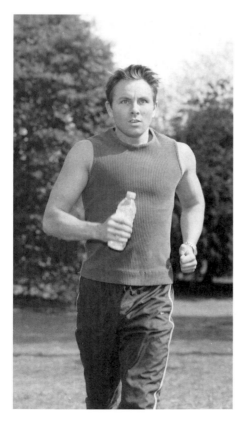

☆ TECHNIQUE TIP ☆
GOOD RUNNING STYLE

Most coaches say that it's not possible to make huge changes to your natural running style (which explains why some top athletes have very individual quirks!). But there are a few principles to bear in mind that will improve your performance:

★ Keep your shoulders down and relaxed and your neck extended and relaxed – neck and shoulder tension is a common problem among runners as they unconsciously scrunch up their shoulders.

★ Try to keep your arms and hands relaxed and by your sides – they shouldn't cross your body as you run.

★ Keep arm swinging to a minimum until you need to sprint – then use the pumping action to increase your speed.

★ Keep your torso upright and your stomach muscles held in.

★ Don't 'sink into your hips' with each step – think 'tall' and 'long'.

★ Land on your heels and roll through your whole foot, taking off from the toes.

★ Don't try to artificially lengthen your stride – you can make faster progress by increasing the number of short strides.

★ Remember to breathe in through your nose and out through your mouth, otherwise you may feel faint.

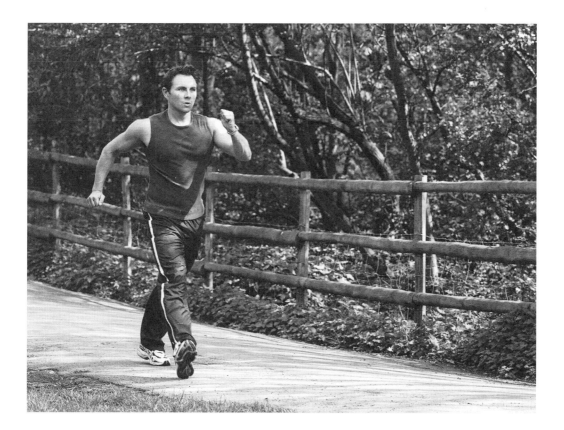

GOAL	COMPLETED
30-min powerwalk/jog	
Front squats 10–15–20–15–10	
Lunges 10–15–20–15–10	
Calf raises 10–15–20–15–10	
Step-ups 10–15–20–15–10	
Straight-leg dead lifts 10–15–20–15–10	
Effort level	
Energy	
Enjoyment	
Overall performance	
COMMENTS:	

FOOD LOG	
FOOD EATEN	**TIME EATEN**
Estimated water consumption	

COMMENTS:

WEEK 1 – DAY 6

This is the last workout day of your first week's training. You have achieved a lot – keep it up! Ignore the negative comments of others – that's their problem.

AM – PYRAMID POWERWALK/JOG

This is it – big effort, focus and overcome.

PM – UPPER BODY POWER CIRCUIT

Maximum effort for maximum results.

FOOD LOG	
FOOD EATEN	**TIME EATEN**
Estimated water consumption	
COMMENTS:	

GOAL	COMPLETED
30-min powerwalk/jog	
Press-ups 5–8–15–8–5	
Bentover row 5–8–15–8–5	
Shoulder press 5–8–15–8–5	
Bicep curls 5–8–15–8–5	
Tricep dips 5–8–15–8–5	
Effort level	
Energy	
Enjoyment	
Overall performance	
COMMENTS:	

WEEK 1 – DAY 7

ACTIVE REST DAY

This is your free day to allow your body time to recover fully. But it doesn't mean you can slob out on the sofa – a short period of moderate activity will help your body recover while reinforcing the gains you've made this week. But moderate is the key – don't do more than 1 hour and keep the intensity level down. If you play a sport such as football or baseball, have a game and you may notice that your hard work throughout the week is already paying off in improved performance. Alternatively, go for a social-based activity such as tennis, hill walking or cycling – getting into the habit of basing part of your social life around active pursuits will help you maintain the results you get from this program in the long term. Your active rest day can also be used as an antidote to a stressful week if you choose a yoga or tai chi class or go swimming.

Choosing What to Eat

Today is also your free day for eating. Taking a more relaxed approach on one day of the week will make sure you don't feel deprived the rest of the time. This is the day to treat yourself to lunch or dinner out with friends or family, have a beer or a glass of wine or enjoy your favourite ice cream. You have worked hard all week and you deserve a reward. Again, as with your exercise, moderation is the key – if you spend all day gorging yourself, you'll undo all your hard work. Bear in mind that eating 3,500 calories over and above your daily needs will result in your body storing a pound of fat. And it is not hard to eat 3,500 calories in one sitting in many restaurants if you go for full-fat, large-sized starters, main course and desserts. Bear these tips in mind:

★ Opt for 2 courses only – starter and main, or main and dessert.
★ If you want a blow-out dessert, order a starter for your main course.
★ Don't consume the contents of the bread basket before your food arrives – get your waiter to take it away if necessary.
★ Keep alcoholic drinks to a minimum.

★ Try to include 2 portions of vegetables in your main meal and, if possible, some fruit in your dessert.

★ Relax, enjoy and feel content with your achievements so far.

☆ TIP OF THE DAY ☆ REASONS TO GIVE UP SMOKING

If you're a smoker, there's never been a better time to give up. You'll get much better results from this program if you give it your best shot. If you smoke, you'll be operating on a reduced lung capacity.

Following an intensive 4-week program naturally requires some lifestyle changes – you can't train twice a day if you spend every evening in the pub. Most smokers find it hardest to give up the cigarettes they have with a drink, so now is the ideal time to give up both. After 4 weeks, you should be over the worst of the cravings and feel less tempted to start smoking again if you do take up your old social life again. If you need more motivation, remind yourself of the facts:

★ Smokers under the age of 50 are five times more likely to die of coronary heart disease than non-smokers, because many of the 4,000 chemicals in tobacco smoke accelerate the furring-up process. As well as this, the carbon monoxide in tobacco smoke deprives the heart of oxygen which can lead to damage and, in the long term, heart failure.

★ We all know there is a well-established link between smoking and lung cancer, but did you know that smokers are also two-thirds more likely to get bladder cancer, twice as likely to get cancer of the kidneys, and six times as likely to develop oral cancers? Half of all cigarette smokers will eventually be killed by tobacco if they don't stop. Smokers who stop in middle age avoid most of the later risk of being killed by tobacco, and those who stop before middle age avoid nearly all the risk.

WEEK 2 TRAINING PROGRAM

	Day 1	Day 2	Day 3
AM	Powerwalk/Jog	Powerwalk/Jog	Powerwalk/Jog
PM	Upper Body Power Circuit	Lower Body Power Circuit	Rest and Recovery

Day 4	Day 5	Day 6	Day 7
Rest and Recovery	Powerwalk/Jog	Powerwalk/Jog	**ACTIVE REST DAY**
Upper Body Power Circuit	Lower Body Power Circuit	Upper Body Power Circuit	

WEEK 2 – DAY 1

You are well rested from your day off. Why not try a new route for your morning work-out so you stay mentally fresh too?

AM – PYRAMID POWERWALK/JOG

PM – UPPER BODY POWER CIRCUIT

PM – UPPER BODY POWER CIRCUIT

This week, for your Power Circuit you have the option of doing your weight work on machines in a gym. If you've never used weight-training equipment before, *it is essential* that you ask a gym instructor to show you the correct way to use the machines before you start.

Barbell and dumbbell options are also included if you prefer to carry on working out at home. It is all effective and the choice is yours. Choose a weight that allows you to complete 12 bicep curls with good technique but no more – the last 2 repetitions should be challenging. It is very important that you get in tune with your body and your individual muscles.

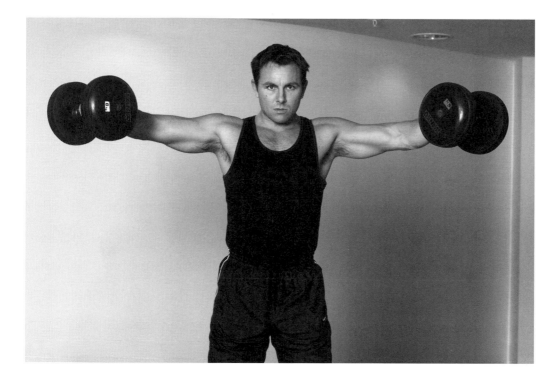

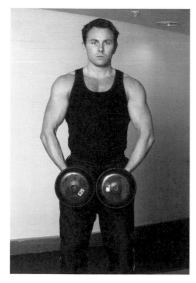

Lateral Raise

In the gym/At home

Stand with your feet hip-width apart, holding a dumb-bell in each hand (heavy enough to allow you to complete 12 repetitions with good technique – but no more). Your hands should face each other. Raise the dumbbells out to the sides, at the same time turning your hands so that they face the floor (as if you were pouring water from a jug). Raise them until your elbows and hands are level with your shoulders (keep your elbows bent). Slowly return to the starting position, resisting the weight on the way down.

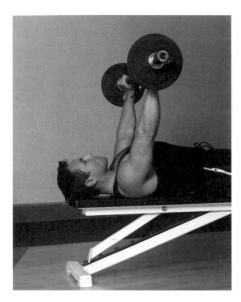 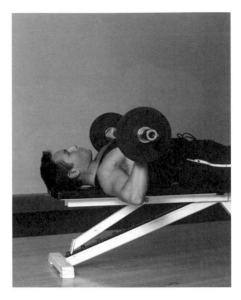

Bench Press

In the gym

Lie on your back on a flat bench, ideally with an attached barbell rack. Attach weights to the barbell that allow you to do 12 repetitions with good technique and no more. Hold the bar with your hands just over shoulder-width apart, palms facing forwards. Remove the bar from the barbell rack and position it directly over your chest with your arms fully extended. Bend your arms, allowing your elbows to travel out to the sides, and slowly lower the bar down to your chest. The bar should touch your upper chest just above the nipple line. Push the bar back to the starting position without locking out your elbows – this will keep the tension on your chest.

At home

Lie on your back on a flat or incline bench. Hold a pair of dumbbells with your palms facing forwards and your arms fully extended, positioned directly over your chest. Slowly lower the dumbbells down to your armpit area. Hold the position for a moment then press the dumbbells back to the starting position without locking out.

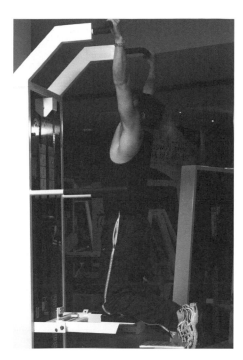
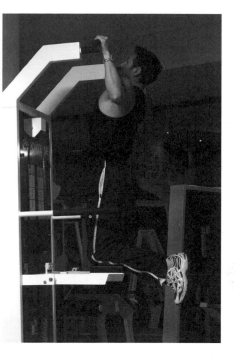

Pull-ups

In the gym

Use a pull-up machine that has a platform to support your weight. Hold the bars above your head with an overhand grip, so your hands are just wider than shoulder-width apart. Your knees should be bent and resting on the platform beneath you. Pull your body up until your eyes are level with the bar. Hold for 1 second then slowly lower yourself back down to the starting position. It is important to isolate your back muscle and squeeze it at the top for optimum contraction.

Bentover row

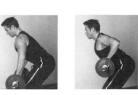

At home

Stand with your feet shoulder-width apart, knees slightly bent. Bend forwards, holding the barbell down in front of your shins. Pull the barbell up to your chest by bending your arms and squeezing your shoulder blades together. Hold for 2 seconds then return to the start position. Squeeze the back muscle.

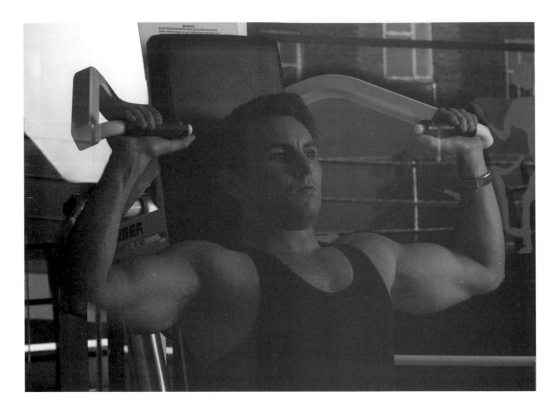

Shoulder press

In the gym

Sit on the shoulder press machine so your back is straight and your lower back is supported. Sit with your feet hip-width apart, gripping the bars with your arms bent at 90 degrees. Press your arms upwards, straightening them but not locking out your elbows. Hold for 1 second then return to the start position. If you struggle, ensure that you push through your heels so you don't arch your back.

At home

Sit on a bench or chair with your back well supported. Hold a weight in each hand with your arms bent at 90 degrees and your elbows out at shoulder level. Press the weights upwards, raising your arms above your head until they are straight but not locked out. Hold for 1 second then return to the start position.

Bicep curls

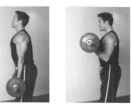

In the gym/at home

Stand with your feet hip-width apart and knees soft. Start with your arms by your sides, elbows slightly bent, holding the barbell in front of you so your palms face away from your body. Slowly raise the barbell to your chest, keeping your elbows tucked in close to your body. Squeeze your biceps then return to the start position.

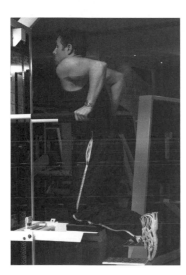

Full dips

In the gym

Using the same dip machine as above, this time place your hands on the parallel bars by your sides with your arms straight and your knees bent and resting on the platform beneath you. Bend your arms, keeping your elbows close to your sides, and slowly lower yourself down until your elbows make an angle of 90 degrees. Pause for a moment then slowly straighten your arms. Don't lean forwards, but feel the pressure through your triceps, focus and isolate.

Full press-ups

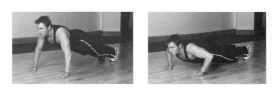

At home

Start with your hands directly under your shoulders, your fingers pointing forwards and your legs straight out behind you. Bend your arms to about 90 degrees and lower your body, keeping your head in line with your spine, and your stomach muscles held in. Lower yourself so your chest is just a couple of inches from the floor. Breathe out and push yourself up to the start position.

Half press-up

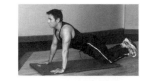

At home

Complete the press-up as above but with your knees resting on the floor throughout.
Top Tip: ensure that you always breathe out on exertion.

How to do the upper body power circuit

Follow a circuit format again, but this time you'll complete only 3. Do the exercises in the order specified, moving quickly from one exercise to the next, following this sequence:

15 reps of each exercise, 1 minute rest
25 reps of each exercise, 1 minute rest
15 reps of each exercise, 1 minute rest.

FOOD LOG	
FOOD EATEN	**TIME EATEN**
Estimated water consumption	
COMMENTS:	

GOAL	COMPLETED
30-min powerwalk/jog	
Lateral raise 15–25–15	
Bench press 15–25–15	
Pull-ups/bentover row 15–25–15	
Shoulder press 15–25–15	
Bicep curls 15–25–15	
Dips/press-ups 15–25–15	
Effort level	
Energy	
Enjoyment	
Overall performance	

COMMENTS:

WEEK 2 – DAY 2

Fitness is a constant learning curve and although what works for one person may not work for another, everyone can be self-disciplined.

> **AM – PYRAMID POWERWALK/JOG**
>
> **PM – LOWER BODY POWER CIRCUIT**

PM – LOWER BODY POWER CIRCUIT

Again, you have the option of doing your Power Circuit in the gym this week, using different equipment.

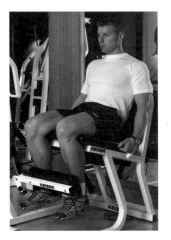 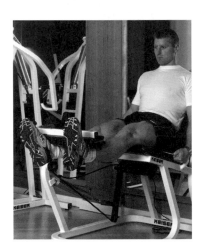

Leg extensions

In the gym

Using the leg extension machine, sit so your thighs are fully supported on the seat – you may have to adjust the seat position. Hook your feet under the roller pads and, holding on to the sides of the seat for balance, slowly straighten your legs. Hold for 2 seconds then return to the start position. Ensure that your legs are fully extended so that you target the right muscle.

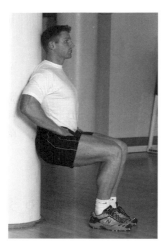

Static squat

At home

Squat next to a wall with your thighs parallel to the floor and the middle of your back against the wall, as if you were sitting on an invisible chair. Hold the position for as long as you can. Do this exercise only once. Feel the burn.

Hamstring curls

In the gym

Lie face down on the leg curl machine and hook your heels under the roller pad. Adjust the machine so that your knees are just off the end of the bench and your thighs are fully supported. Hold on to the handgrips or the edge of the bench, bend your knees and bring your heels towards your backside. Hold for 2 seconds then lower your heels back to the starting position. Don't allow your bottom to rise up but keep your groin pressed into the machine.

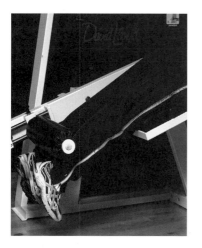
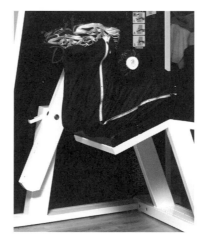

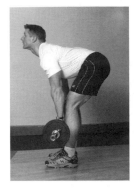

Straight-leg dead lift with barbell

At home

Stand in front of the barbell with your feet parallel and shoulder-width apart. Bend your legs until your hips and knees are at the same level, keeping your rib cage up and your head level. Your back should be straight, at a 45-degree angle to the floor. Grasp the bar with your hands and using the power of your hips and thighs, lift the bar from the floor straightening your legs at the same time. The bar should reach the upper part of your thighs before you slowly return it to the floor.

Standing calf raises

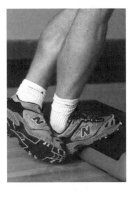

In the gym

Using a standing calf raise machine, place your shoulders under the pads and step on to the block and allow your heels to hang off the edge. Your feet should be hip-width apart and pointing directly ahead. Straighten your legs as you lift the selected weight clear of the rest of the stack. Rise on your toes as high as possible, hold for a count of 2 then slowly lower your heels down as far as they will go. Stretch your calves fully at the bottom of the movement – your heels should be lower than your toes.

At home

Place a barbell across the back of your shoulders and perform the calf raise as above. Stand on a step or block with your heels hanging off to increase the range of movement.

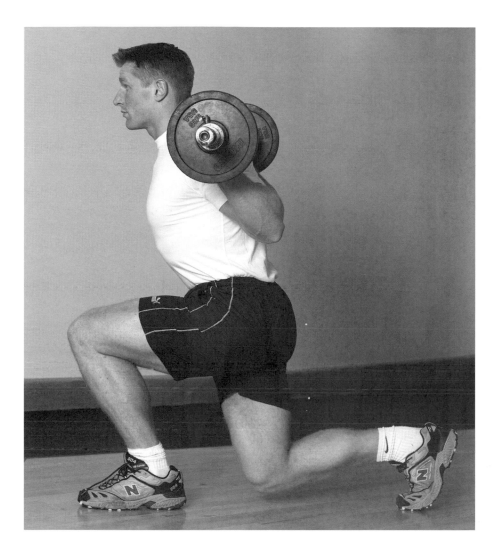

Reverse lunges

In the gym/at home

Stand with your feet shoulder-width apart and your knees soft, holding the barbell across the back of your shoulders. Step back one stride with your right leg, placing the top of your foot on the floor. Lower the knee until it almost touches the floor, hold for 1 second then return to the start position and repeat with the left leg.

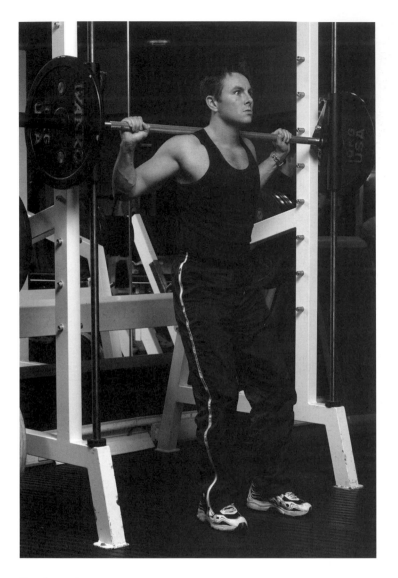

Front squats

In the gym

Using a Smith machine, stand with your feet just over shoulder-width apart directly under the barbell and angled slightly outwards. Place the barbell across the back of your shoulders. Keeping your head up and your trunk erect, slowly bend your legs and lower yourself down until your thighs are parallel to the ground. Straighten your legs by pushing hard through your heels until you return to the start position.

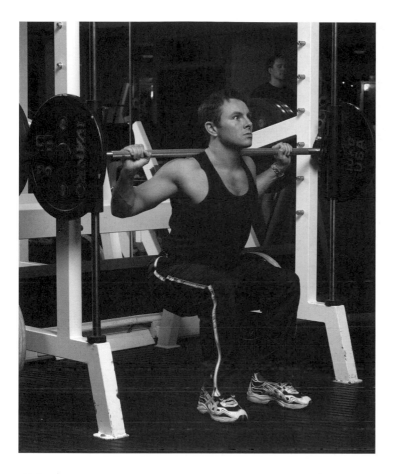

At home

Do the exercise as above with a barbell on your shoulders.

DOING THE LOWER BODY POWER CIRCUIT

Do the exercises in the order specified, moving quickly from one exercise to the next, following this sequence, keeping up the intensity:

   10 reps of each exercise, 1 minute rest
   15 reps of each exercise, 1 minute rest
   25 reps of each exercise, 1 minute rest
   15 reps of each exercise, 1 minute rest
   10 reps of each exercise, 1 minute rest.

GOAL	COMPLETED
30 min powerwalk/jog	
Leg extensions/static squat 10–15–25–15–10	
Hamstring curls/ straight-leg dead lift 10–15–25–15–10	
Standing calf raises 10–15–25–15–10	
Reverse lunges 10–15–25–15–10	
Front squats 10–15–25–15–10	
Effort level	
Energy	
Enjoyment	
Overall performance	
COMMENTS:	

★ Remember to complete your food log for the day.

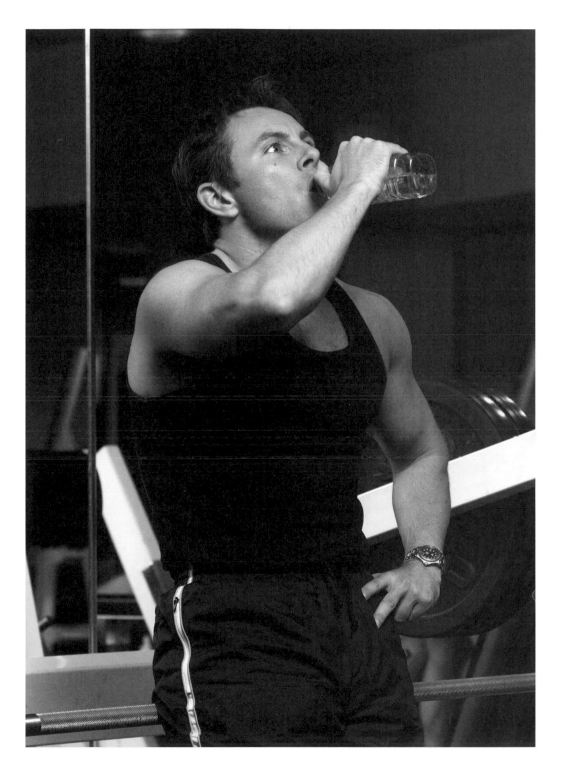

WEEK 2 – DAY 3

Refresh your motivation by rereading Chapter 2.

> **AM – PYRAMID POWERWALK/JOG**
>
> **PM – REST AND RECOVERY**

☆ TECHNIQUE TIP ☆ WHAT A CUP OF COFFEE CAN DO FOR YOU

If you need a boost to get you through your exercise session, drink a cup of coffee. In studies, caffeine has been shown to improve the performance of endurance athletes by up to 20%, partly by increasing blood circulation and dilation of the airways in the lungs. It also has an effect on the brain which makes you perceive exercise as less intense.

Caffeine consumption has also been shown to lead to a temporary increase in the metabolism and the rate of fat breakdown. Caffeine helps free up the triglycerides stored in the adipose tissues, which are broken down into fatty acids to be released into the bloodstream and used as fuel. This is an old favourite of endurance athletes who want to use fat as fuel and preserve precious stores of glycogen (sugar found in the muscles) as long as possible.

The International Olympic Committee allows athletes to compete with an upper level of 20mg of caffeine per litre of blood, which translates at around 5–6 cups of normal strength coffee in 1–2 hours. It is not a good idea to make this a regular habit – a couple of cups of coffee an hour before a long run or session at the gym can make it feel a lot easier, but relying on any substance to boost your performance is something I discourage. If you feel it is really essential, then a milky coffee it has to be. And, as caffeine is a diuretic, be sure to drink water to keep you hydrated throughout your session.

GOAL	COMPLETED
30-min powerwalk/jog	
Effort level	
Energy	
Enjoyment	
Overall performance	
COMMENTS:	

★ Remember to complete your food log for the day.

WEEK 2 – DAY 4

> **AM – REST AND RECOVERY**
>
> **PM – UPPER BODY POWER CIRCUIT**

☆ **TIP OF THE DAY** ☆
4 REASONS TO THROW AWAY YOUR BATHROOM SCALES

★ Most are inaccurate anyway.
★ If you want to lose weight, it is fat loss that counts. Muscle weighs more than fat so even if you're dropping fat, you may weigh more on the scales if you're strength training regularly.
★ Your weight can fluctuate on a daily basis depending on how hydrated you are.
★ A tape measure is a far more accurate way to record your changing body composition.

★ Remember to complete your food log for the day.

GOAL	COMPLETED
Lateral raise 15–25–15	
Bench press 15–25–15	
Pull-ups/bentover row 15–25–15	
Shoulder press 15–25–15	
Bicep curls 15–25–15	
Dips/press-ups 15–25–15	
Effort level	
Energy	
Enjoyment	
Overall performance	
COMMENTS:	

WEEK 2 – DAY 5

AM – PYRAMID POWERWALK/JOG

PM – LOWER BODY POWER CIRCUIT

☆ TECHNIQUE TIP ☆ GO SLOW WITH WEIGHTS

Although time is at a premium for most of us, don't be tempted to rush through your reps to get your weight training over and done with. The faster you go, the more momentum you will use rather than your own muscles – and that means the less effect you get from each exercise. Slow, controlled movements are also more effective because they allow you to use correct technique. This means that you are more likely to isolate and work only the required muscle, rather than engaging the surrounding connecting muscles. During a typical repetition, the contraction (when the muscle works) should last about 2 seconds and the elongation (when it relaxes) about 3 seconds.

★ Remember to complete your food log for the day.

GOAL	COMPLETED
30 min powerwalk/jog	
Leg extensions/static squat 10–15–25–15–10	
Hamstring curls/ straight-leg dead lift 10–15–25–15–10	
Standing calf raises 10–15–25–15–10	
Reverse lunges 10–15–25–15–10	
Front squats 10–15–25–15–10	
Effort level	
Energy	
Enjoyment	
Overall performance	
COMMENTS:	

WEEK 2 – DAY 6

You're very nearly halfway through the program now. If you find your initial enthusiasm starting to wane, don't let that get in the way of doing the work. You'll have highs and lows throughout this program but keep your goals in mind, stick to your plan and you'll get there.

AM – PYRAMID POWERWALK/JOG

PM – UPPER BODY POWER CIRCUIT

☆ **TECHNIQUE TIP** ☆ **PUT YOUR MIND BEHIND YOUR MUSCLE**

Recent research has shown that if you *think* about a specific muscle as you work it, you'll see bigger increases in strength than if you do the same exercise with your mind elsewhere. It may sound unlikely, but it makes sense when you consider that muscles move in response to impulses from nearby motor neurons and the firing of those neurons depends on the strength of impulses sent by the brain. So whatever exercise you're doing, focus your mind on the muscle you're working – try to think of it contracting then relaxing.

★ Remember to complete your food log for the day.

GOAL	COMPLETED
30 min powerwalk/jog	
Lateral raise 15–25–15	
Bench press 15–25–15	
Pull-ups/bentover row 15–25–15	
Shoulder press 15–25–15	
Bicep curls 15–25–15	
Dips/press-ups 15–25–15	
Effort level	
Energy	
Enjoyment	
Overall performance	
COMMENTS:	

WEEK 2 – DAY 7

ACTIVE REST DAY

Two weeks completed and you deserve some rest! Today is your active rest day.

Today is also the ideal day to do the Basic Fitness Test again and see how much you've improved. Don't forget to record your results (*see* pages 55–57).

BASIC FITNESS TEST (2)

This is it – time to test yourself! So focus, motivate yourself, put on that music and go for it. Good luck.

Measurements

Use a tape measure to record the circumference of your chest, upper arm, waist, hips and upper thigh.

Sit-ups

Record how many basic crunches you can do with good slow technique until you can do no more (*see* page 74 for how to do the perfect crunch).

Press-ups

Record how many full or half press-ups you can do with good technique (*see* pages 83–84 for how to do the perfect press-up).

Standing jump test

Stand next to a wall with chalk on your fingers. Bend your knees and jump as high as you can, touching the wall at your highest point. Record the measurement.

Recovery

Powerwalk for 1½ miles or for 15 minutes. Run back or alternate run/walk. Rest for 30 seconds then take your pulse for 6 seconds. Times the result by 10. This is your recovery heart rate (*see* page 56).

	★ Test 1 ★ Date:	★ Test 2 ★ Date:	★ Test 3 ★ Date:
Chest measurement			
Arm measurement			
Waist measurement			
Hip measurement			
Thigh measurement			
Number of sit-ups			
Number of press-ups			
Standing jump test			
Recovery heart rate			

WEEK 3 TRAINING PROGRAM

	Day 1	Day 2	Day 3
AM	Powerwalk/Jog	Powerwalk/Jog	Powerwalk/Jog
PM	Upper Body Power Circuit	Lower Body Power Circuit	Rest and Recovery

Day 4	Day 5	Day 6	Day 7
Rest and Recovery	Powerwalk/Jog	Powerwalk/Jog	ACTIVE REST DAY
Upper Body Power Circuit	Lower Body Power Circuit	Upper Body Power Circuit	

WEEK 3 – DAY 1

Now you're into Week 3 you should be starting to consolidate your training. You are on familiar ground now and will be finding out about how your body is responding to the work. It's time to really get stuck in to the meat of the program.

AM – PYRAMID POWERWALK/JOG

PM – UPPER BODY POWER CIRCUIT

☆ **TECHNIQUE TIP** ☆ **DON'T FORGET YOUR AB WORK**

Are you fitting in 3 sessions of ab work a week? If you find you're too tired or pushed for time to do them after a workout, then try doing them first. After all, when you consider just how important the abdominal muscles are, it seems crazy to spend only the very last 5 minutes of a workout focusing on them. Start your workout with your ab exercises, and you'll not only do them with better form, but you're also more likely to hold your abs in tight for the rest of the session, which means they are getting a workout as well.

★ Remember to complete your food log for the day.

GOAL	COMPLETED
30 min powerwalk/jog	
Lateral raise 15–25–15	
Bench press 15–25–15	
Pull-ups/bentover row 15–25–15	
Shoulder press 15–25–15	
Bicep curls 15–25–15	
Dips/press-ups 15–25–15	
Effort level	
Energy	
Enjoyment	
Overall performance	
COMMENTS:	

WEEK 3 – DAY 2

> **AM – PYRAMID POWERWALK/JOG**
>
> **PM – LOWER BODY POWER CIRCUIT**

☆ TIP OF THE DAY ☆ USE A TRAINING DIARY

Have you completed all of your workouts so far? Although you have two 'AWOL' cards that you can use if you have to miss a workout during the 4 weeks, remember that missing any more than this will mean that the program won't be as effective and you won't get the best from it. Use a training diary if you are finding it difficult to find time for the workouts. Writing down your training plans for the next seven days at the beginning of a week will make it easier to plan the rest of your life around the workouts and means that you are more likely to stick to the program.

★ Remember to complete your food log for the day.

GOAL	COMPLETED
30 min powerwalk/jog	
Leg extensions/ static squat 10–15–25–15–10	
Hamstring curls/ Straight–leg dead lift 10–15–25–15–10	
Standing calf raises 10–15–25–15–10	
Reverse lunges 10–15–25–15–10	
Front squats 10–15–25–15–10	
Effort level	
Energy	
Enjoyment	
Overall performance	
COMMENTS:	

WEEK 3 – DAY 3

AM – PYRAMID POWERWALK/JOG
PM – REST AND RECOVERY

GOAL	COMPLETED
30-min powerwalk/jog	
Effort level	
Energy	
Enjoyment	
Overall performance	
COMMENTS:	

☆ TECHNIQUE TIP ☆ IMAGE THERAPY

If you are trying to change your behaviour, then pick up some healthy habits or drop some less useful ones. Don't simply make mental lists of tasks of things such as *'I must stop eating cake/drinking beer.'* Instead, think *'Who do I want to become?'* Is the sort of person you want to be strong, fit, healthy and full of energy? Then think, *'What actions would this person take? What would they eat, how would they deal with stress, how would they start each day?'* Focus on developing yourself, rather than changing what you are doing.

★ Remember to complete your food log for the day.

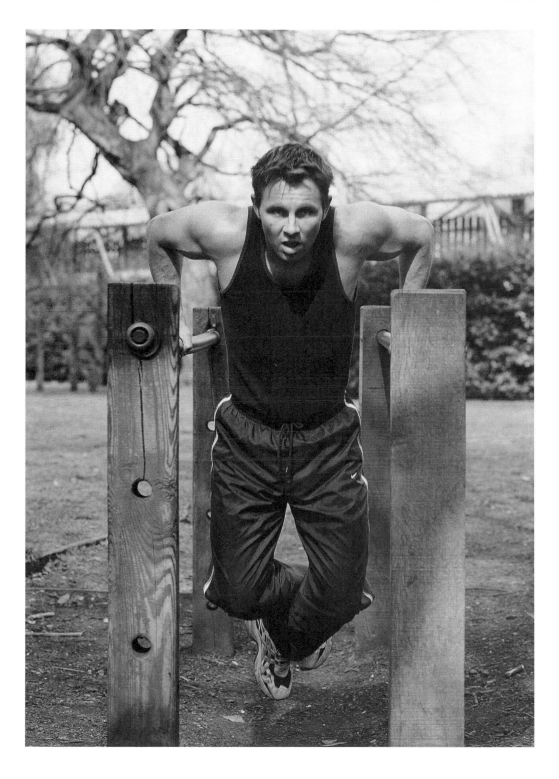

WEEK 3 – DAY 4

AM – REST AND RECOVERY

PM – UPPER BODY POWER CIRCUIT

☆ TIP OF THE DAY ☆ LEARN TO READ FOOD LABELS

The bulk of your food plan on your 30-day program should be made up of fresh, unprocessed food. But some of the food you eat will inevitably be of the packaged variety – unless you can afford a personal chef to prepare dishes from scratch every day. It is not a crime to buy packaged food – just learn to decipher the labels so you can buy the healthiest. Here's what to look for:

★ **List of ingredients.** This must be stated in descending order of weight (the heaviest listed first, the lightest last). Whatever comes first in the list of ingredients is what there is most of. So, if 'hydrogenated oil' is the first item listed, this means it is loaded with saturated fat and should go straight back on the supermarket shelf

★ **Fat content.** Claims like 'low fat' or 'lower fat' can be misleading (low-fat potato chips, for instance, are still a high-fat product). Check how many grams of fat a product contains and bear in mind that you should not be eating more than 40g a day if you are female or 60g a day if you are male

★ **Additives.** Don't be fooled by claims such as 'no artificial flavours' – it could have artificial preservatives or colours! Look for foods that omit all three.

★ Remember to complete your food log for the day.

GOAL	COMPLETED
30 min powerwalk/jog	
Lateral raises 15–25–15	
Bench press 15–25–15	
Pulls-ups/bentover row 15–25–15	
Shoulder press 15–25–15	
Bicep curls 15–25–15	
Dips/press-ups 15–25–15	
Effort level	
Energy	
Enjoyment	
Overall performance	
COMMENTS:	

WEEK 3 – DAY 5

AM – PYRAMID POWERWALK/JOG

PM – LOWER BODY POWER CIRCUIT

☆ **TIP OF THE DAY** ☆

Keep up an intake of at least 3–5 pieces of fruit a day. As well as all the vitamins and minerals, fruit contains the sugar fructose which will give you extra energy.

★ Remember to complete your food log for the day.

GOAL	COMPLETED
30 min powerwalk/jog	
Leg extensions/ static squat 10–15–25–15–10	
Hamstring curls/ straight-leg dead lift 10–15–25–15–10	
Standing calf raises 10–15–25–15–10	
Reverse lunges 10–15–25–15–10	
Front squats 10–15–25–15–10	
Effort level	
Energy	
Enjoyment	
Overall performance	
COMMENTS:	

WEEK 3 – DAY 6

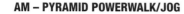

AM – PYRAMID POWERWALK/JOG

PM – UPPER BODY POWER CIRCUIT

☆ TIP OF THE DAY ☆ YOUR DAILY WORKOUT RECORD

You're nearly in the last week of your 4-week workout and it's important to focus on pushing yourself right up to the last day of the workout, using your exercise time effectively and watching your diet. An easy way to motivate yourself is to look back over your daily workout records from the first 10 days and see how far you have progressed in just a short time. You can also use the records to check for any weak areas – look at whether you are completing most workouts and if you are working at the right intensity.

★ Remember to complete your food log for the day.

GOAL	COMPLETED
30 min powerwalk/jog	
Lateral raises 15–25–15	
Bench press 15–25–15	
Pulls-ups/bentover row 15–25–15	
Shoulder press 15–25–15	
Bicep curls 15–25–15	
Dips/press-ups 15–25–15	
Effort level	
Energy	
Enjoyment	
Overall performance	
COMMENTS:	

WEEK 3 – DAY 7

If you've been doing your best for 3 weeks now, you're probably feeling that things have changed, mentally and physically. Areas of muscle will be firmer, your lungs will be opening up and you are more alert – and you are closer to your goals.

ACTIVE REST DAY

☆ TIP OF THE DAY ☆ MAKE EVERY DAY AN ACTIVE DAY

Following a fitness program is the best way to get in shape. But to give yourself the best possible chance of maintaining this fitness in the long term, you need to look at your lifestyle. Your workouts account for around 7 hours activity a week. That leaves 161 hours when you're not working out! What you do in those hours will make the difference between whether you live your life as a fit, lean person or an overweight sedentary one. You may have read a million times that you should 'take the stairs instead of the elevator'. You probably just dismissed it – how can it make a difference? True, running up the stairs once won't make any difference at all. But choosing the stairs in preference to the elevator every day of your life will. Activity and movement has a cumulative effect – the more active you are throughout the day, the fitter your body becomes. The following are suggestions how you can make this a part of your life:

★ Walk, don't ride, whenever you can
★ Lose your TV remote control so you have to get up to change channels
★ At work, get up from your desk and walk around every 20 minutes
★ Plan your social events around active hobbies rather than eating and drinking.

★ Remember to complete your food log for the day.

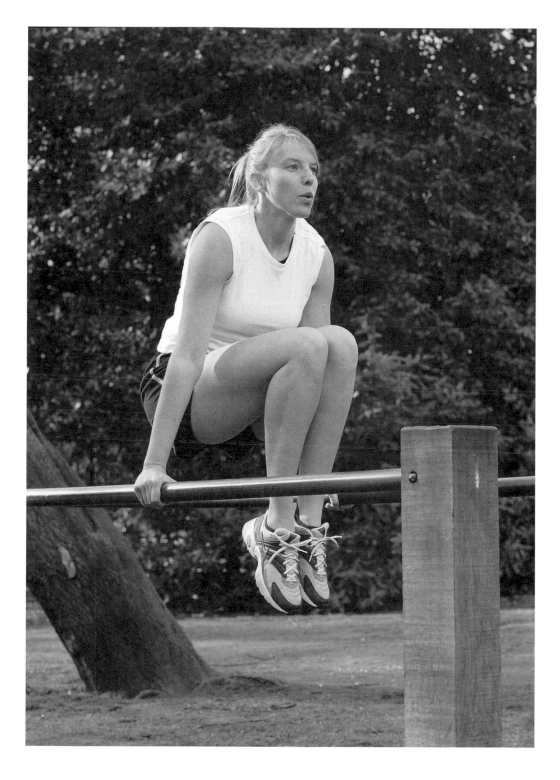

WEEK 4 TRAINING PROGRAM

	Day 1	Day 2	Day 3
AM	Cardio Power Circuit	Rest and Recovery	Cardio Power Circuit
PM	Rest and Recovery	Top-to-Toe Plyometric Circuit	Rest and Recovery

Day 4	Day 5	Day 6	Day 7
Rest and Recovery	Cardio Power Circuit	Rest and Recovery	PROGRAM COMPLETED
Top-to-Toe Plyometric Circuit	Rest and Recovery	Top-to-Toe Plyometric Circuit	

WEEK 4 – DAY 1

The final week of the program and you are now ready to crank up the intensity of your cardio work.

AM – CARDIO POWER CIRCUIT

Equipment needed: Adjustable bench (set horizontal) or a park bench if you want to work outdoors.

PM – REST AND RECOVERY

AM – CARDIO POWER CIRCUIT

The Cardio Power Circuit will work your heart and lungs as well as challenging muscle strength and endurance at the same time. Apart from the alternate squat thrust, you've done all of these exercises before, so there's no reason not to do your best work this week. The 3 sets of this circuit bring together the moves you have practised in a fast-moving sequence that will keep your heart rate elevated.

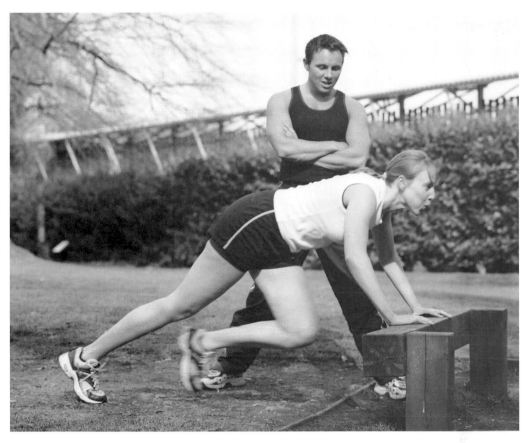

Alternate squat thrusts

Start with your hands on the bench and your feet straight out behind you. Bend one leg and bring it up so the knee is below your chest and your weight is resting on the ball of the foot. Straighten the leg again as you bend the other leg. Repeat as fast as possible but keep the form.

In Set 2, do the same action with your hands on the floor.

DOING CARDIO POWER CIRCUIT

Start off with a 5-minute warm-up of walking or slow jogging. Then complete the following circuit at a steady pace with no rests between exercises. Complete the circuit once then cool down with 5 minutes of walking, followed by Full Body Stretches (*see* pages 70–72).

Set 1

10 Tricep dips

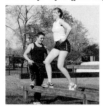

10 Step-ups (per leg)

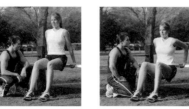

10 Press-ups (hands on bench)

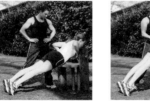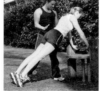

10 Reverse lunges

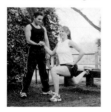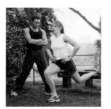

10 Alternate squat thrusts (hands on bench)

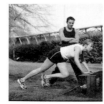

Set 2

15 Tricep dips

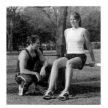 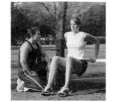

15 Step-ups (per leg)

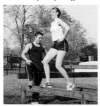

15 Press-ups (hands on bench)

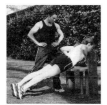 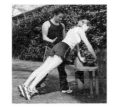

15 Reverse lunges

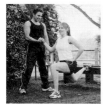 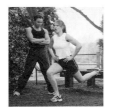

15 Alternate squat thrusts (hands on the floor)

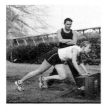

Set 3 (see images in Set 1)

10 Tricep dips

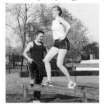

10 Step-ups (per leg)

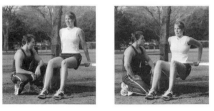

10 Press-ups (hands on bench)

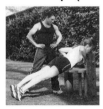 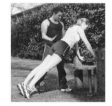

10 Reverse lunges

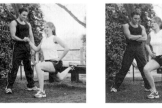 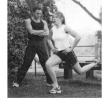

10 Alternate squat thrusts (hands on bench)

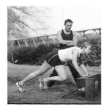

PM – REST AND RECOVERY

GOAL	COMPLETED
30-min powerwalk/jog	
Tricep dips 10–15–10	
Step-ups (per leg) 10–15–10	
Press-ups 10–15–10	
Reverse lunges 10–15–10	
Squat thrusts 10–15–10	
Effort level	
Energy	
Enjoyment	
Overall performance	
COMMENTS:	

★ Remember to complete your food log for the day.

WEEK 4 – DAY 2

This new 'plyometric' circuit adds a new dimension to your basic body resistance workout. Every muscle in the body is used when you work with the barbell and dumbbells, but this time there's also the addition of plyometric exercises to build specifically on your 'fast twitch' muscle power. Plyometrics are explosive movements that are guaranteed to challenge and develop your muscle power. But be warned – they're tough. You've got 3-minute rests between circuits and you will definitely need them!

AM – REST AND RECOVERY

PM – TOP-TO-TOE PLYOMETRIC CIRCUIT

Equipment needed: Barbell, dumbbells, adjustable bench (set horizontal)

Cleans with barbell

Stand in front of the barbell with your feet parallel and shoulder-width apart. Bend your legs until your hips and knees are at the same level, keeping your rib cage up and your head level. Your back should be straight, at a 45-degree angle to the floor. Grasp the bar with your hands just over shoulder-width apart and, using the power of your legs and hips, lift the bar from floor and straighten your legs at the same time. Then bend your legs slightly and lift the bar over your head, holding for 1 second before reversing the movement until the barbell is back at your feet. Keep your back straight and the bar as close as possible to your body throughout the movement.

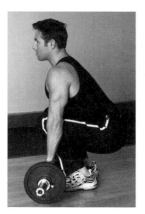
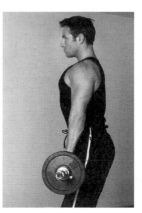
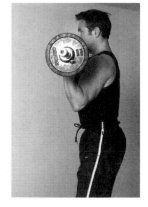

Alternate squat thrusts

As before (*see* page 159).

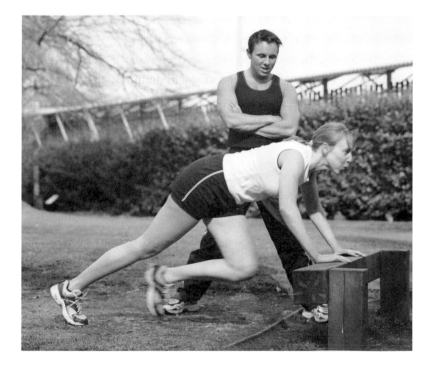

Press-ups

As before (*see* page 83).

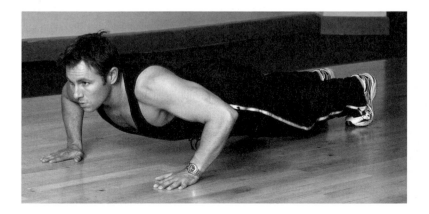

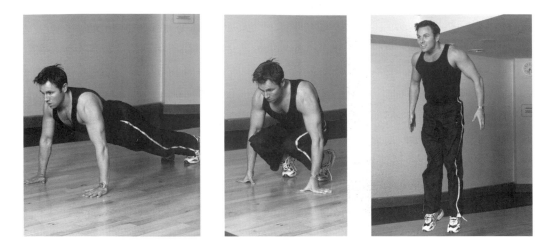

Burpees

Start by standing upright, with feet together and knees soft. Drop down to a crouch position with your hands on the floor in front of you. Jump your legs backwards so you end up in a full press-up position. Jump your legs forwards again to the crouch position. Jump up to standing position and jump on the spot so that your feet leave the ground.

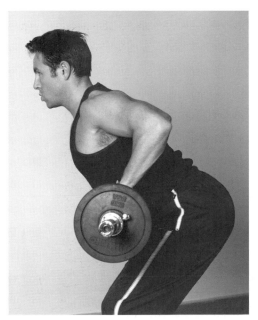

Bentover rows

As before (*see* page 84).

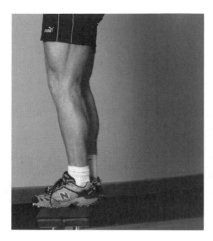

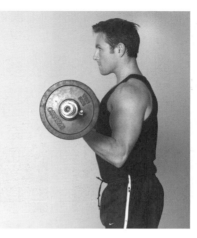

Step-ups

As before (*see* page 92).

Bicep curls

As before (*see* page 86).

Burpees

Complete as above but omit the final jump in the standing position.

Tricep dips

With your hands shoulder-width apart on a chair or bench and your legs straight out in front of you, bend your elbows to 90 degrees and then raise yourself back to your original position.

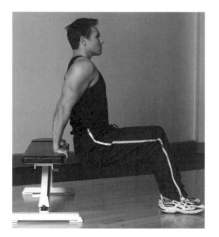

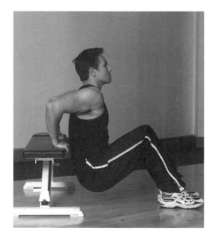

Sumo wide-leg squats

Stand with your feet just over shoulder-width apart and your toes angled outwards at about 45 degrees. Hold the barbell so it rests on your upper back. Keeping your head up and your trunk erect, slowly bend your legs and squat down. Lower yourself until your thighs are parallel to the floor. Straighten your legs by pushing hard through the heels and repeat.

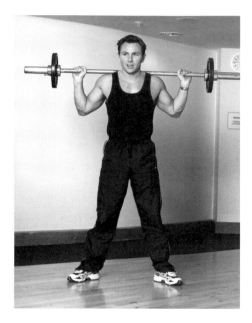 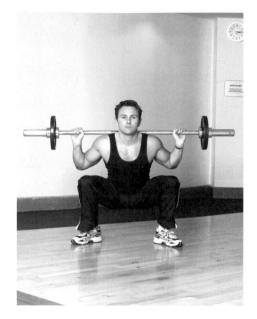

DOING THE TOP-TO-TOE PLYOMETRIC CIRCUIT

Do the exercises in the order specified, moving quickly from one exercise to the next, following this sequence:

    10 reps of each exercise, 3 minutes rest
    15 reps of each exercise, 3 minutes rest
    8 reps of each exercise, full body stretches.

★ Remember to complete your food log for the day.

GOAL		COMPLETED
Cleans with barbell 10–15–8		
Alternate squat thrusts 10–15–8		
Press-ups 10–15–8		
Burpees 10–15–8		
Bentover rows 10–15–8		
Step-ups 10–15–8		
Bicep curls 10–15–8		
Burpees 10–15–8		
Tricep dips 10–15–8		
Sumo wide-leg squats 10–15–8		
Effort level		
Energy		
Enjoyment		
Overall performance		
COMMENTS:		

WEEK 4 – DAY 3

AM – CARDIO POWER CIRCUIT

PM – REST AND RECOVERY

☆ **TECHNIQUE TIP** ☆
3 WAYS TO GET YOURSELF TO THE GYM WHEN YOU REALLY DON'T FEEL LIKE IT

★ Tell yourself that you'll go and sit in the sauna. Chances are, you'll do your workout when you get to the gym.

★ Tell yourself you'll only do 10 minutes of your workout. Chances are you'll do the whole thing once you get started.

★ If you have a permanent locker, always leave something in it that you'll need very soon – such as your watch or an important work file. You'll be forced to go to the gym again soon to pick it up.

★   Remember to complete your food log for the day.

GOAL	COMPLETED
Tricep dips 10–15–10	
Step-ups (per leg) 10–15–10	
Press-ups 10–15–10	
Reverse lunges 10–15–10	
Squat thrusts 10–15–10	
Effort level	
Energy	
Enjoyment	
Overall performance	
COMMENTS:	

WEEK 4 – DAY 4

AM – REST AND RECOVERY
PM – TOP-TO-TOE PLYOMETRIC CIRCUIT

GOAL		COMPLETED
Cleans with barbell 10–15–8		
Alternate squat thrusts 10–15–8		
Press-ups 10–15–8		
Burpees 10–15–8		
Bentover rows 10–15–8		
Step-ups 10–15–8		
Bicep curls 10–15–8		

Burpees 10–15–8		
Tricep dips 10–15–8		
Wide-leg squats 10–15–8		
Effort level	
Energy	
Enjoyment	
Overall performance	
COMMENTS:	

★ Remember to complete your food log for the day.

WEEK 4 – DAY 5

AM – CARDIO POWER CIRCUIT	
PM – REST AND RECOVERY	

GOAL	COMPLETED
Tricep dips 10–15–10 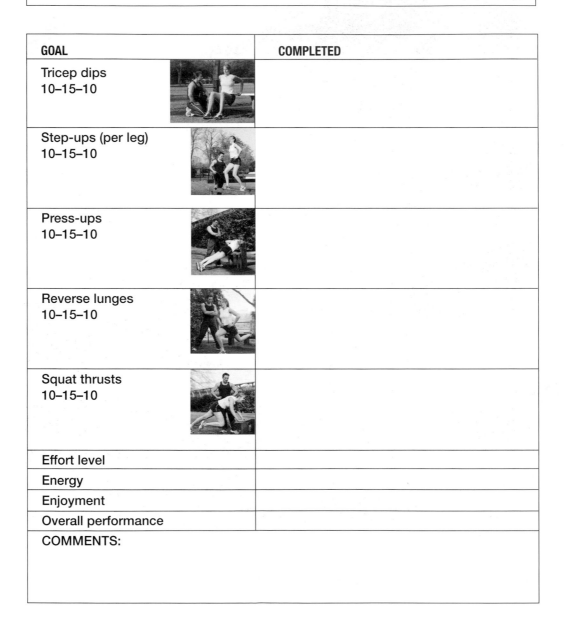	
Step-ups (per leg) 10–15–10	
Press-ups 10–15–10	
Reverse lunges 10–15–10	
Squat thrusts 10–15–10	
Effort level	
Energy	
Enjoyment	
Overall performance	
COMMENTS:	

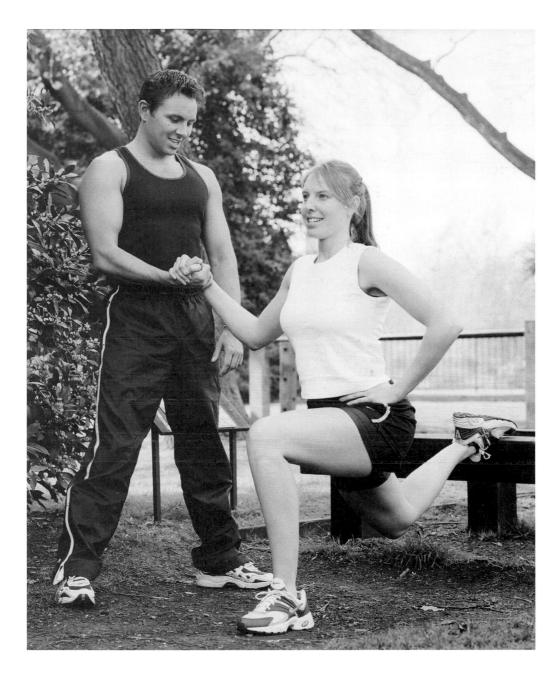

★ Remember to complete your food log for the day.

WEEK 4 – DAY 6

You are nearing the end of what's been a tough but rewarding experience. You have had the opportunity to test yourself – both mentally and physically – and I hope you are aware that you have done something special. This is the last workout day of the Commando Workout program, so do yourself proud and make it your best day yet.

As you complete your final workout of the program, now would be a good time to look at the changes you have made to your lifestyle to accommodate this exercise regime and to think about how you can continue to include the workouts in your daily life and to review your eating habits in the long-term.

AM – REST AND RECOVERY

PM – TOP-TO-TOE PLYOMETRIC CIRCUIT

★ Remember to complete your food log for the day.

GOAL		COMPLETED
Cleans with barbell 10–15–8		
Alternate squat thrusts 10–15–8		
Press-ups 10–15–8		
Burpees 10–15–8		
Bentover rows 10–15–8		
Step-ups 10–15–8		
Bicep curls 10–15–8		
Burpees 10–15–8		
Tricep dips 10–15–8		
Wide-leg squats 10–15–8		
Effort level		
Energy		
Enjoyment		
Overall performance		
COMMENTS:		

WEEK 4 – DAY 7

THE END – OR JUST THE BEGINNING!

Congratulations – you have reached the end of the Commando Workout. You've come a long way, you have a lot to be proud of and now you can reap the rewards. Your lung capacity is greater than before; your heart is in better shape than before; your body fat percentage should be lower than before, and your stamina levels should be far higher now. All that work also means that your body shape has changed – you are now likely to be more toned and showing greater muscle definition. But most important is the self-discipline and focus that you have displayed to get you through the program. If you can take the mental stamina that you have developed and apply it to your everyday life, tasks will seem just so much easier. Now you have learnt these mental lessons there is no harm in challenging yourself. Life is full of challenges, but to a hero like you they will be so much simpler to overcome.

So, there is only one task left to do – your third and final Basic Fitness Test. Record your results (*see* pages 55–57) and see what a difference you have made.

Although this program lasts 4 weeks, your life goes on. If you have enjoyed making a change and discovering new personal strengths along the way, you don't have to stop now. You have shown you can have the discipline and motivation to keep yourself in shape – so take it on board and start planning your next challenge … Some additional information on this can be found at the end of this book (*see* Moving On, page 182).

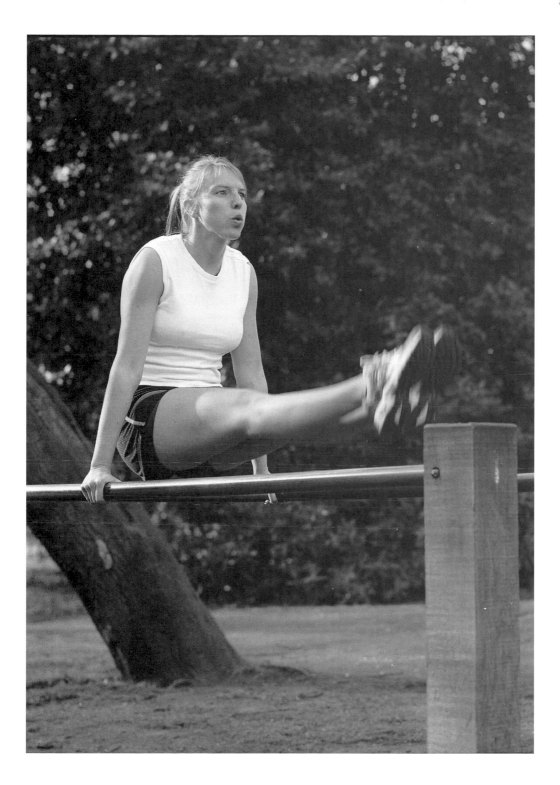

BASIC FITNESS TEST (3)

Measurements

Use a tape measure to record the circumference of your chest, upper arm, waist, hips and upper thigh.

Sit-ups

Record how many basic crunches you can do with good slow technique until you can do no more (*see* page 74 for how to do the perfect crunch).

Push-ups

Record how many full or half push-ups you can do with good technique (*see* pages 83–84 for how to do the perfect push-up).

Recovery

Powerwalk for 1½ miles or for 15 minutes. Run back or alternate run/walk. Rest for 30 seconds then take your pulse for 6 seconds. Times the result by 10. This is your recovery heart rate.

Standing jump test

Stand next to a wall with chalk on your fingers. Bend your knees and jump as high as you can, touching the wall at your highest point. Record the measurement.

	★ Test 1 ★ Date:	★ Test 2 ★ Date:	★ Test 3 ★ Date:
Chest measurement			
Arm measurement			
Waist measurement			
Hip measurement			
Thigh measurement			
Number of sit-ups			
Number of push-ups			
Standing jump test			
Recovery heart rate			

MOVING ON

During your 4-week program you have become familiar with several different styles of workout. Maintaining and improving on your fitness level is as simple as mixing and matching these workouts. But bear in mind the following principles:

★ Aim to complete 3 cardiovascular sessions (30-minute Pyramid Powerwalk/Jog or 30-minute Cardio Power Circuit) each week
★ Aim to complete both an upper body and a lower body circuit at least once a week
★ Never work the same muscle groups 2 days in a row. In other words, always do an upper body circuit the day after a lower body circuit rather than 2 lower body circuits in a row
★ Always allow at least one complete rest day a week
★ Use your personal exertion rates to ensure you are continually challenging your body – ask yourself, are you really pushing yourself to level 9 with every workout?
★ Don't forget to do your ab workouts 3 times a week
★ Re-read chapter 2 whenever you find your motivation waning.

It's a good idea to give yourself an occasional break from training. Apart from the possibility of suffering from the symptoms of overtraining (*see* page 43), we all need a break now and again. Try to split up your workouts into 4-week blocks and this will help you maintain the focus and motivation to achieve the goals you set yourself. And remember, make your goals realistic ones so they don't become barriers you can't overcome. Above all, enjoy yourself!

Please feel free to register your results and give any feedback on my website:

WWW.SIMONWATERSON.COM

Best wishes and good luck!

RESOURCES

UK

Fitness Industry Association (UK)
115 Eastbourne Mews
Paddington
London
W2 6LQ
Tel: 020 7298 6730
Fax: 020 7298 6731
E-mail: info@fia.org.uk
Website: www.fia.org.uk

David Lloyd Leisure Ltd
The Arena
Parkway West
Cranford Lane
Hounslow
Middlesex
TW5 9QΛ
Tel: 020 8564 6600
Website: www.davidlloydleisure.co.uk

British Journal of Sports Medicine
BMJ Publishing Group
BMA House
Tavistock Square
London
WC1H 9JR
Website: sss.bjsm.bmjjournals.com

Premier Global Ltd
Premier House
Willowside Park
Canal Road
Trowbridge
Wiltshire
BA14 8RH
Tel: 01225 353 535
Website: www.premierglobal.co.uk

Simon Waterson studied to become a personal trainer with Premier Training International. Premier Global provides products and services to the health and fitness industry and is the leading provider of training for personal trainers. Premier Training International, our specialized training arm, trains personal trainers from all backgrounds and offers bespoke packages for those still serving in the British armed forces, and a resettlement package for those whose service career has come to an end.

For more information log onto www.premierglobal.co.uk or for a free copy of the training prospectus, please call 01225 353535.

USA

American Council on Exercise (ACE)
4851 Paramount Drive
San Diego
California 92123
Tel: (858) 279 8227 or (800) 825-3636
Fax: (858) 279 8064
Website: www.acefitness.com

American College of Sports Medicine
401 W. Michigan St.
Indianapolis
IN 46202-3233
Tel: (317) 637 9200
Fax: (317) 634 7817
Website: www.acsm.org

The Simon Waterson Fit Kit

This unique 'fit kit' is your own personal trainer. As the military take essential kit with them everywhere they go, the Simon Waterson Fit Kit holds basic fitness and workout items that can be used in a variety of different ways. Designed to be taken on holiday, to the office or to the park, it is perfect for people who want to take their workout wherever they go.

This stylish, compact backpack contains:
★ Interchangable dumbbells
★ Skipping rope
★ Resistance band with handles
★ Dynoband
★ Stopwatch
★ Waterbottle
★ Sweatband and neck towel
★ Specially designed workout cards designed by Simon Waterson

A fantastic gift for anyone about to embark on an exercise plan or for anyone who takes their personal fitness seriously, the Simon Waterson Fit Kit can be ordered from my website: www.simonwaterson.com.

Thank you, keep fit and, most of all, have fun.

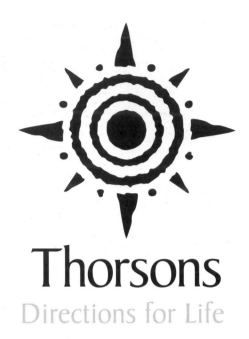

Thorsons

Directions for Life

www.thorsons.com

This online sanctuary is packed with information, inspiration and guidance to help you on the path to physical and spiritual well-being. Drawing on the integrity and vision of our authors and titles, and with health advice, articles, astrology, tarot, a meditation zone, author interviews and events listings, Thorsons.com is a great alternative to help create space and peace in our lives.

So if you've always wondered about practising yoga, following an allergy-free diet, using the tarot or getting a life coach, we can point you in the right direction.

Make www.thorsons.com your online sanctuary.